The Paleo Beginners Guide

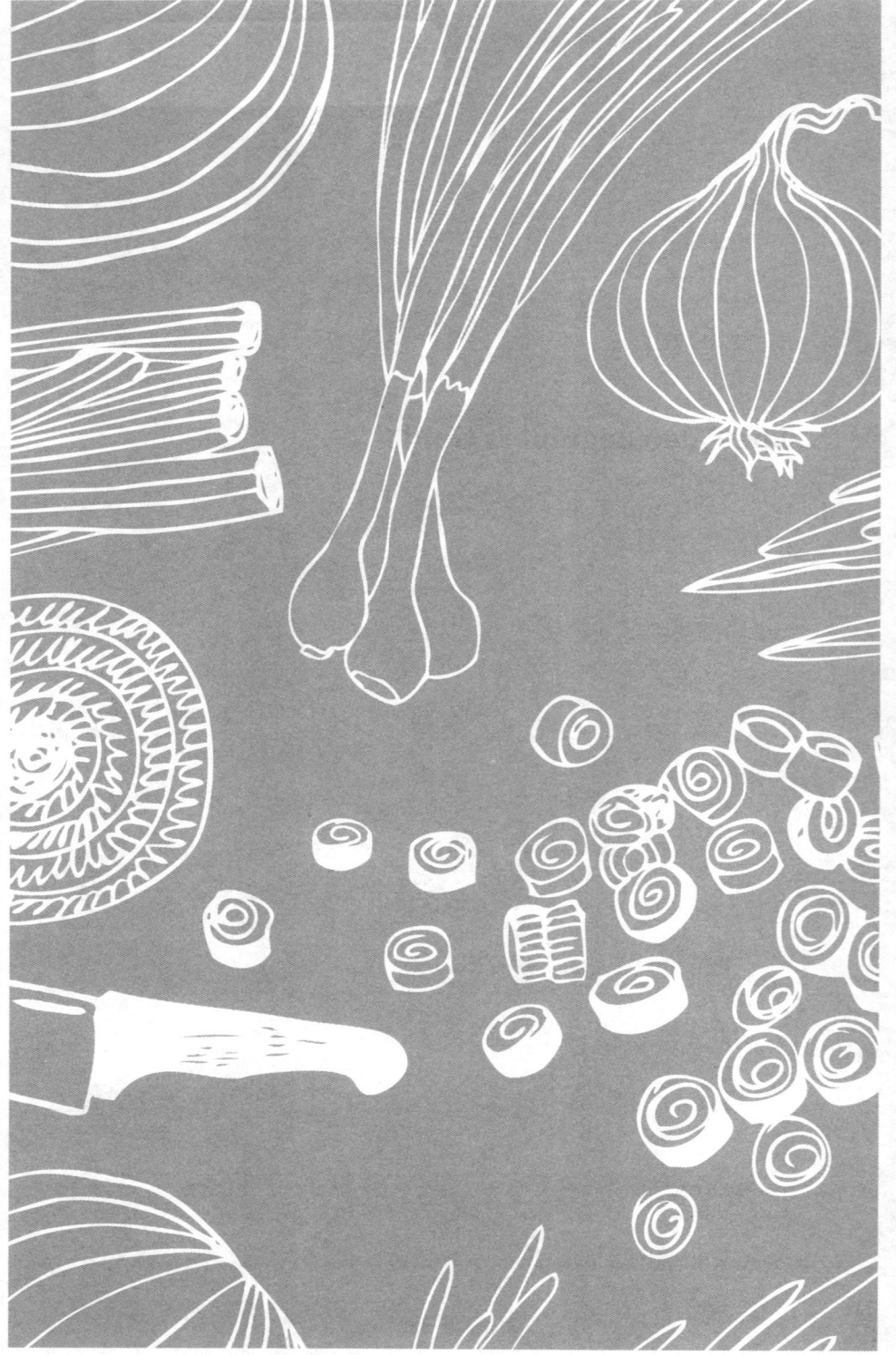

The Paleo Beginners Guide

A SPECIAL EDITION OF THE *NEW YORK TIMES* BEST SELLER *PALEO FOR EVERY DAY*

Presented by Dr. Ryan Lazarus

No part of this publication may be reproduced, stored in a retrieval system, or transmitted in any form or by any means, electronic, mechanical, photocopying, recording, scanning, or otherwise, except as permitted under Section 107 or 108 of the 1976 United States Copyright Act, without the prior written permission of the publisher.

Limit of Liability/Disclaimer of Warranty: The publisher and the author make no representations or warranties with respect to the accuracy or completeness of the contents of this work and specifically disclaim all warranties, including without limitation warranties of fitness for a particular purpose. No warranty may be created or extended by sales or promotional materials. The advice and strategies contained herein may not be suitable for every situation. This work is sold with the understanding that the publisher is not engaged in rendering medical, legal, or other professional advice or services. If professional assistance is required, the services of a competent professional person should be sought. Neither the publisher nor the author shall be liable for damages arising herefrom. The fact that an individual, organization, or website is referred to in this work as a citation and/or potential source of further information does not mean that the author or the publisher endorses the information the individual, organization, or website may provide or recommendations they/it may make. Further, readers should be aware that Internet websites listed in this work may have changed or disappeared between when this work was written and when it is read.

Contents

Introduction   1

PART ONE

Getting Started

Chapter One: Paleo Diet Basics   5

Chapter Two: How to Use the Paleo Diet Meal Plan   25

PART TWO

Putting the Paleo Diet Meal Plan into Action

Chapter Three: Week One   39

Chapter Four: Week Two   47

Chapter Five: Week Three   55

PART THREE

Paleo Diet Recipes

Chapter Six: Breakfast   65

Chapter Seven: Lunch   89

Chapter Eight: Dinner   107

Chapter Nine: Dessert   137

Chapter Ten: Pantry Recipes   155

Appendix: Paleo Snacks   167

Resources   169

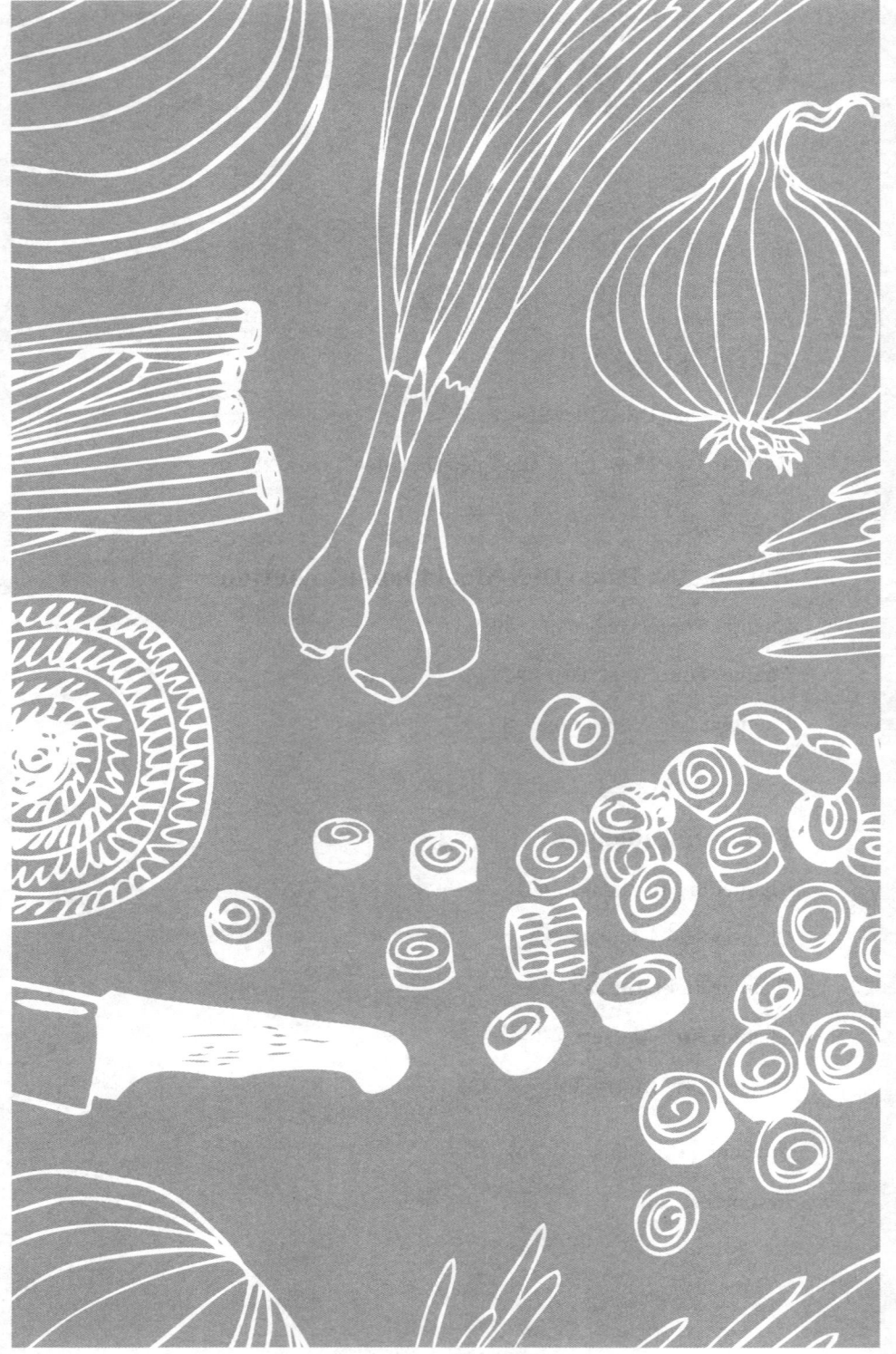

Introduction

The *Paleo Beginners Guide* was created to detoxify your body, burn fat, and build lean muscle. Following this plan, you'll transform your body, boost your nutritional intake, and improve your overall health.

More specifically, this meal plan balances your hormones for effective and sustainable weight loss. It helps stabilize your brain chemistry for increased clarity of thought. It improves endocrine health and metabolic functionality, and promotes digestive health and more complete nutrient absorption. It even helps reduce and manage stress. And it helps you sleep more soundly.

After just a few days of eating a Paleo diet, it will be clear why so many people follow the Paleo way of eating and living. In this book, you'll find a simple-to-follow twenty-one-day meal program with easy recipes for breakfast, lunch, dinner, dessert, and quick snacks. Each week starts off with a detailed shopping list to help you save both time and money. Daily tips, cooking terms, guidelines, and other motivators will help you stay on the Paleo plan and be successful with it.

The Paleo lifestyle delivers noticeable results without leaving you feeling starved or deprived. *The Paleo Beginners Guide* is the plan to get you started on the way to a new, improved you.

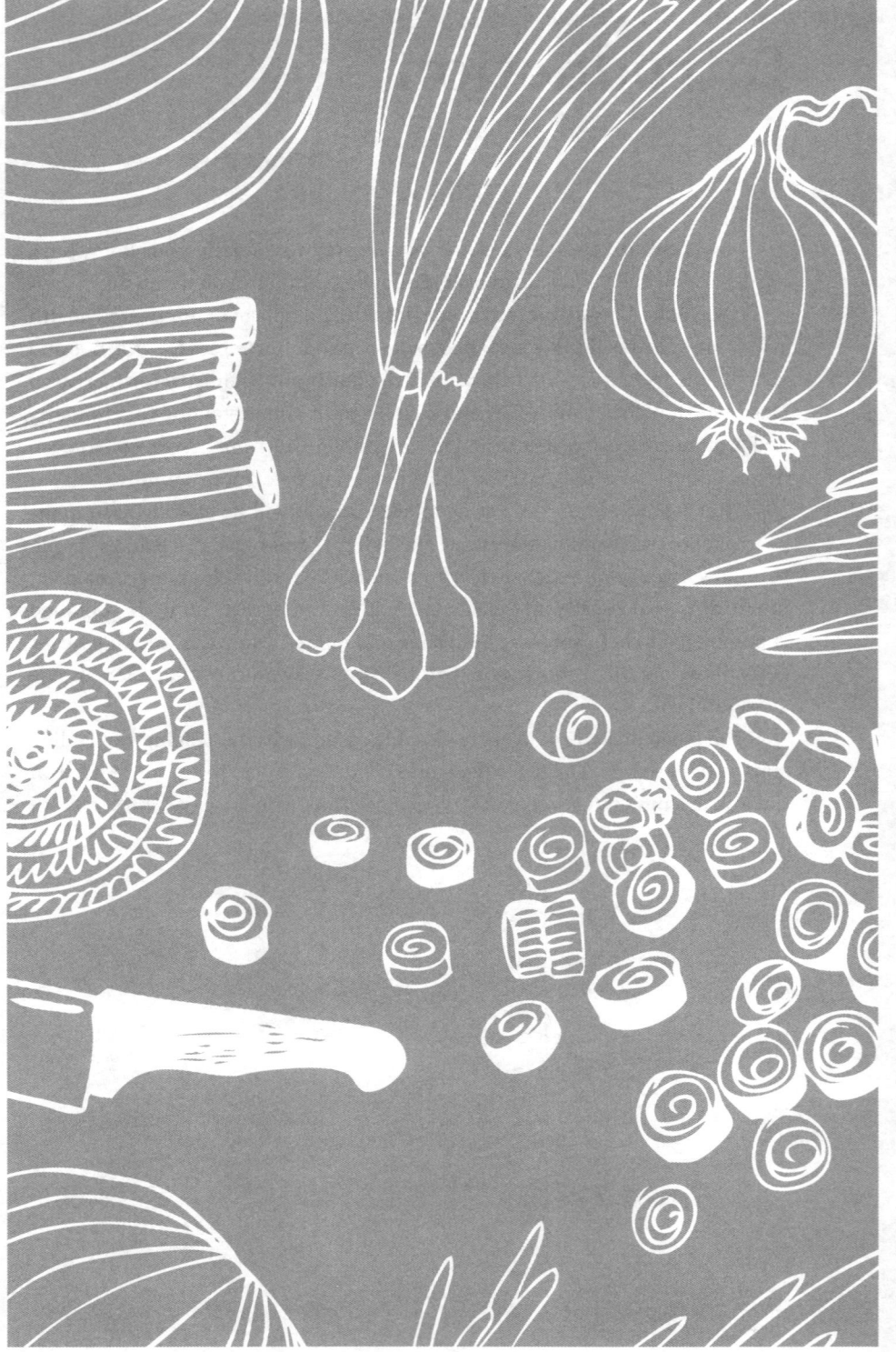

PART ONE

Getting Started

CHAPTER ONE PALEO DIET BASICS

CHAPTER TWO HOW TO USE THE PALEO DIET MEAL PLAN

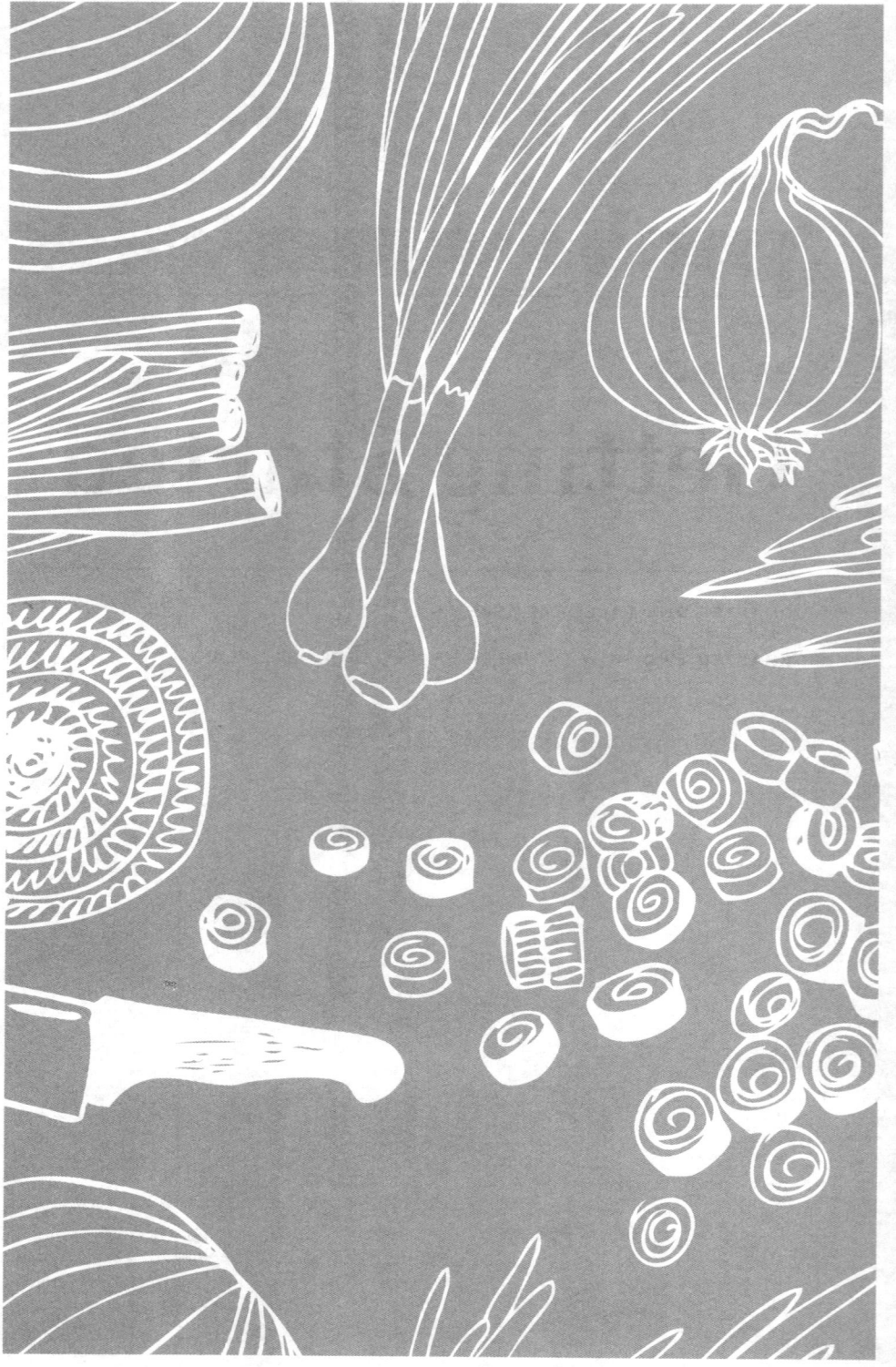

CHAPTER ONE

Paleo Diet Basics

Paleo is a way of life. The name and concept of the Paleo lifestyle is based on the idea of eating what our human ancestors subsisted on during the Paleolithic era. Our ancestors were hunters and gatherers who ate only what they could harvest, fish, hunt, or scavenge. Paleo followers believe that our bodies were designed to eat as these early people did, and doing so will enable us to remain healthy, muscular, and fit.

Paleo nutritionists and many other scientists believe that evolution has not caught up with the advances of our society. By consuming the foods that sustained our ancestors (such as pastured meats, sustainable seafood, fresh vegetables, wild fruit, and foraged nuts) rather than those produced by modern agricultural and commercial processing methods (such as grains, legumes, dairy, sugars, and artificial additives), we can maximize nutrition absorption and burn foods more efficiently. In the long run, experts believe, eating the Paleo way will stave off harmful diseases and improve overall health and well-being.

Unlike other high-protein, low-carb diets, eating the Paleo way focuses on feeding your body the best-quality, most sustainably produced, least processed foods possible. When it comes to carbohydrates, the Paleo lifestyle encourages consuming only low-glycemic carbs from fresh vegetables along with fruits that are low in sugar to stabilize and maintain insulin levels. Quality protein from wild-caught seafood and pastured meat and eggs—rather than from commercially produced or processed proteins—repairs and builds muscle. And eating omega-3 fatty acids found in grass-fed meat, seafood, and nuts and seeds promotes better heart and brain health.

While the Paleo lifestyle encourages you to prepare more of your meals at home, you also have many options when dining out. But once you start using *The Paleo Beginners Guide*'s shopping, cooking, and food storage tips, you'll see how easy this "cleaner," healthier way of eating can be. And how much better you look and feel.

PALEO LIFESTYLE GUIDELINES

As we've pointed out, the Paleo lifestyle focuses on consuming nutritious vegetables and fruits along with quality proteins and fats. To make the most of the Paleo plan, it's important to avoid refined sugars, dairy, grains, and processed foods with added sodium, preservatives, and other unnatural ingredients.

Here's a quick look at some of the foods you will enjoy on the Paleo diet:

- Healthful oils and fats
- Hormone- and antibiotic-free meat (preferably from pasture-raised, grass-fed animals)
- Most fruits, with an emphasis on berries
- Most vegetables
- Nuts and seeds
- Sustainably sourced fish and shellfish

Here are the main groups of foods you will avoid when eating Paleo:

- Added salt
- Dairy
- Grains and legumes
- Hydrogenated and other processed oils (sunflower, canola)
- Partially hydrogenated oils (margarine, alternative butter spreads)
- Processed foods
- Refined and artificial sugars

The Paleo lifestyle does not involve calorie counting. Instead, you eat Paleo-approved foods when you're hungry and stop when you're satisfied. The meal plans show you how to balance every meal and snack with lean proteins, healthful fats, and vegetables and/or fruits. Still, this isn't a license to go crazy. Stick to the recommended portion sizes. If you're still hungry, incorporate an additional Paleo-friendly snack to your day or increase your vegetable and protein portions.

WHY FOLLOW THE PALEO DIET?

Current nutritional research links diseases like type 2 diabetes, heart diseases, autoimmune disorders, and even some cancers with eating too many processed foods, sugars, saturated fats, and refined carbohydrates—the unfortunate staples of the modern American diet.

Avoiding the disease-causing foods and eating the Paleo diet has many benefits:

- Clearer skin and healthier hair, nails, and teeth
- Fat loss and improved muscle tone
- Improved digestion and reduced allergies and food sensitivities
- Increased energy
- More efficient workouts
- Reduced inflammation throughout the body
- Reduced risk of long-term diseases, such as heart disease, hypertension, and diabetes
- Stabilized blood sugar

Anti-inflammation. Repeated studies have shown that refined and processed foods, grains, and dairy can increase inflammation in the body that may cause the immune system to mistake healthy cells for disease-causing pathogens and attack them. Some believe there is a strong link between chronic bodily inflammation and many forms of cancers and autoimmune diseases. The Paleo way of eating focuses on avoiding foods that may cause inflammation and instead eating antioxidant-rich vegetables and fruits that promote healthy cell production, swallow up cancer-causing free radicals, and boost our bodies' illness-fighting capabilities. Fruits and vegetables are also slightly alkaline, which means they help reduce acidity in the body, another known culprit for certain diseases and energy deprivation.

Heart health. Paleo encourages the consumption of omega-3 fatty acids, which are shown to lower bad cholesterol levels and boost the good, improve blood chemistry, and boost brain health. Some studies suggest that we ingest too many omega-6 fats, commonly found in processed foods and refined oils, and that this may contribute to chronic inflammation, impeding the absorption of heart-healthy nutrients. Even some olive oils, which are thought to be healthful, are overly processed and stripped of their nutritional properties. If we raise the level of omega-3 fatty acids in our bodies by eating more foods rich in omega-3s and limiting omega-6 fats, we can improve the health of our hearts and minds.

Recent clinical studies have shown that high-protein diets are more effective in improving cholesterol than low-fat, high-carbohydrate diets. This is because the body burns proteins and fats more efficiently than it does sugars and excess carbohydrates, which convert to and are stored as fat when not burned off, leading to weight gain as well as increased "bad" cholesterol levels and potentially heart disease in the long run.

Improved digestion. Some refined and processed foods like gluten and dairy have been linked to poor digestion issues and in some cases, may even cause damage to the intestinal lining. This damage can allow undigested foods and toxins to flow back into the bloodstream and cause "leaky gut" syndrome, which can lead to food sensitivities and allergies, chronic inflammation, and other long-term health problems. The Paleo diet removes processed and refined foods from the menu, helping you avoid or recover from these problems.

Hormone stabilization. Eating Paleo has been shown to improve hormone levels in the body. When hormone levels are out of balance, they can impede weight loss and lead to other problems, like excess body fat, low energy levels, high stress, and problems with blood sugar. For example, when cortisol, also known as the "stress" hormone, is out of balance, it can cause the body to store excess fat and slow metabolism.

Hypertension prevention. The Paleo way of eating naturally reduces your salt intake, which can help prevent bloating and even help reduce blood pressure. Many processed foods, dairy products, and restaurant meals contain high amounts of sodium that may easily put you over your daily limit. Eating more whole foods and cooking your own meals helps prevent hypertension in the long run. Though you will find salt as an ingredient in some of the recipes in this book, the amounts are low; the type of salt used is important, too. Look for mineral-rich sea salts rather than table and kosher salts, which are processed. You'll also be seasoning your meals with healthful fats, chili peppers, herbs, lemon juice, and other acids to boost flavor, so you won't miss the excess salt.

Most adults should not consume more than 2,300 mg of sodium per day, the amount found in just 1 teaspoon of table salt. According to the American Heart Association, ideally we should ingest no more than 1,500 mg of sodium per day, and we need a daily dose of only 200 mg to survive.

THE PALEO LIFESTYLE AND WEIGHT LOSS

The Paleo lifestyle is very different from other eating plans and "diets." While weight loss may happen when eating the Paleo way, people may also see a noticeable drop in their body fat.

Paleo eating, combined with regular cardio and strength-training exercise, will literally change your body shape. You'll feel and look leaner, stronger, and more toned. Many find they lose more stomach fat eating this way, as well.

We now also know that eating fat doesn't make you fat. Scientists say protein and fat burn two to three times faster than carbohydrates. Starchy carbs and sugars do not burn as effectively and convert to fat faster, which can impede metabolism and lead to long-term weight gain.

In addition, eating more protein, healthful fats, and "good" carbohydrates, rather than loading up on starchy carbs and sugars, will keep you satiated longer and potentially even reduce the amount you need to eat, by stabilizing your blood sugar. The key hormone your body uses to stabilize blood sugar is insulin, and excess levels can cause metabolic syndrome, which can lead to obesity, hypertension, cholesterol problems, and type 2 diabetes. As mentioned earlier, cutting back on processed foods and eating more wholesome, nutritious foods can help stabilize hormones, which is also shown to promote weight loss.

Many Paleo lifestyle adopters also exercise regularly to speed up their metabolism as well as reduce stress and improve mental health. Subscribing to a good balance of cardio and strength-training will help your body not only burn calories but also build muscle to burn more fat throughout the day. Changing your exercises every day and incorporating high-intensity interval workouts can help your body burn even more fat. This again has "Paleolithic" implications: Our ancestors had to respond on the fly to sudden danger and be able to shift gears quickly during hunting—no two days of exercise looked the same for people in the Paleolithic era.

Some studies show that shorter, higher-intensity bursts of exercise burn more fat than longer, more sustained cardio workouts like running. Switching up your exercise routine from day to day or week to week can also strengthen more muscles and prevent injuries caused by more repetitive exercises.

PALEO FOODS TO ENJOY

Too many diets place heavy restrictions on foods you can't eat, which leads to cravings and hunger, dissatisfaction and frustration. While certain foods are encouraged over others, the Paleo lifestyle is more about making better choices and enjoying fresh, high-quality foods that other eating plans restrict, including: lean proteins; fats like avocados, eggs, and nuts; and sweet treats, too. With so many options and by eating balanced meals, you should never feel deprived. Here's a closer look at the Paleo-approved foods.

Meat and Eggs

- Beef
- Bison
- Chicken
- Eggs
- Lamb
- Pork

The meat and seafood that our cavemen and women ancestors ate didn't come shrink-wrapped and pumped full of antibiotics, hormones, and added sodium. That's why the Paleo lifestyle encourages choosing grass-fed, pastured meats; wild-caught fish; and wild-caught or farmed shellfish from sustainable, environmentally conscious producers over more commercially produced beef, chicken, pork, and eggs, where animals may have been raised in confined spaces and fed less-than-ideal diets.

For all recipes that call for meat ingredients, assume that free-range, pastured, and antibiotic- and hormone-free are best. Organic does not always mean pastured, but at the very least, it suggests the animal ate a healthier diet. When selecting eggs, look for free-range or pastured ones, which naturally have higher levels of omega-3 fatty acids.

Farmers' markets are the best sources for high-quality proteins, but shopping this way is not always financially or geographically possible. If available, sign up for a share in a community-supported agriculture (CSA) program to buy meat, vegetables, fruits, and eggs in bulk. Some Paleo-supportive gyms and other outlets work directly with local, sustainable farmers to offer such food shares. When shopping at the grocery store, watch out for false claims and always read the labels and ingredient lists carefully (see the "Learn to Read Food Labels" section in Chapter Two).

When purchasing bacon, make sure it is nitrate-free and watch out for the excess use of sugars and salts in the ingredients. Try to select bacon made from pastured, free-range pork.

Sausages and hot dogs often contain excess sodium, nitrates, and other additives. A Paleo-friendly sausage will use natural animal casings and contain good-quality meat, some spices, and minimal amounts of salt.

Seafood

- Arctic char
- Cod, trout, and other whitefish
- Halibut
- Lobster, mussels, oysters, and other shellfish
- Salmon
- Tuna (canned tuna in moderation)

Choose sustainably sourced seafood, which means fish and shellfish that's either wild-caught or farmed using environmentally safe practices. Watch out for seafood coming from countries outside the United States, where many fisheries have come under fire for ocean destruction and poor food handling. Look closely at aquarium "watch lists" to know which seafood is more sustainable than others.

Non-Animal-Based Proteins

Though the Paleo lifestyle discourages dairy, whey-based protein powder is considered acceptable because it does not contain potentially harmful lactose and other acids. Paleo and other nutritionists often suggest avoiding dairy products containing lactose because of the potential gastrointestinal effects on digestion—diarrhea or constipation—and because dairy products have high acidity levels, which have been shown to increase inflammation in the body. Still, not all protein powder is considered equal when following Paleo. When choosing whey-based powders, look for brands made with grass-fed dairy products, and be leery of added sugars, stabilizers, and preservatives. Many natural food stores, Paleo-friendly gyms, and online sites carry these powders.

Hemp seed powder is a good alternative to whey, but some brands have a bitter taste. If you are exercising and lifting weights regularly, supplementing your protein intake with some amino acid powders and blends can be beneficial for muscle building and repair, but again, read labels carefully.

Vegetables

- Alfalfa and other sprouts
- Artichoke
- Asparagus
- Beets
- Bell peppers
- Bok choy
- Broccoli
- Brussels sprouts
- Cabbage
- Carrots
- Cauliflower
- Celery
- Cucumbers
- Eggplant
- Garlic
- Green and yellow beans
- Greens: kale, spinach, Swiss chard, mustard, beet, turnip, watercress
- Jicama
- Kohlrabi
- Leeks
- Lettuces: Bibb, escarole, red leaf, arugula, Belgian endive, romaine
- Mushrooms
- Okra
- Onions and green onions
- Peppers
- Pumpkin
- Radishes
- Rutabaga
- Squash: summer, yellow, spaghetti, butternut*, delicata*
- Sweet potato*
- Tomatoes
- Turnips*
- Zucchini

Note: Vegetables marked with an asterisk (*) should be eaten in moderation because of their higher sugar levels.

When purchasing vegetables, sustainable sources, such as local farmers and markets, are best, but organic is also preferable.

If your budget is too tight to purchase all organic produce, try to at least buy organic for vegetables and fruits with peels or skin you plan to eat rather than remove, such as apples, cucumbers, bell peppers, and in some cases, sweet potatoes. Avocados, lemons, limes, and onions with peels to be removed, for example, can be sourced in the commodity aisle. Once at home, use a natural vegetable wash (with citric acid, not chemicals) to remove waxes that are applied to many fruits and vegetables, including even organic produce. Also, opt for vegetable-storage or mesh bags for enhanced freshness when storing produce in the refrigerator.

Fruits

- Apples
- Blackberries
- Blueberries
- Cherries
- Dried fruits, unsweetened and unsulfured or with no sugar added, such as cherries, cranberries, and blueberries
- Goji berries
- Lemons
- Limes
- Strawberries

Some Paleo purists choose to eat only berries, since they were once the only fruits gathered by our ancestors, but others include additional low-glycemic, high-fiber fruits like apples and cherries. Melons, stone fruits, grapefruit, and oranges in whole, not juice, form are also allowed, but *The Paleo Beginners Guide* excludes those. When adding fruit with higher glycemic indexes to your diet, do so slowly and note your body's response. If you feel a sudden sugar "high" or feel hungrier even after eating some, you may have a low tolerance for these fruits. Watch out for bananas, too, which are starchier and have higher levels of sugar. When eating fruit, have a little protein or healthful fats with it to prevent your blood sugar from spiking.

Consider taking vitamin C supplements in lieu of citrus fruits or juices to help with muscle repair and to boost your immune system. Because vitamin C is a water-soluble vitamin, you don't have to worry about taking too much. Your body will naturally flush out what's not used.

Healthful Fats and Oils

- Almond
- Avocado
- Coconut
- Extra-virgin olive oil
- Flaxseed (unfiltered)
- Grape-seed
- Hazelnut
- Walnut

Choose unrefined oils rather than processed ones when choosing healthful oils. Avocado has also been applauded as a healthful fat, with its high level of vitamin E, which is great for improving skin, hair, and nails. Coconut, once thought to have too much saturated fat, is now accepted as a healthful fat. Choose unrefined coconut oil and unsweetened coconut flakes and meat when selecting this fat.

Some Paleo purists avoid butter altogether, while others eat butter sourced from grass-fed or pastured cows because of its higher omega-3 fat levels. Ghee, a form of butter in which the whey has been removed, is acceptable in some Paleo circles. Like coconut and avocado oils, ghee has a high smoking point, which is great for searing, baking, and high-temperature broiling and roasting. Grape-seed oil also has a high smoking point and a neutral taste, but some Paleo purists find it to be too refined.

Reserve nut oils for salad dressings and flavoring vegetables and other foods after they have been cooked. Nut oils are too delicate to retain their nutritional properties when cooked.

Nuts and Seeds

- Almonds (raw, roasted and unsalted)
- Brazil nuts (raw)
- Chia seeds
- Flaxseeds
- Hazelnuts (raw, roasted and unsalted)
- Macadamia nuts (raw, roasted and unsalted)
- Pistachios (raw, roasted and unsalted)
- Pumpkin seeds
- Sesame seeds
- Sunflower seeds
- Walnuts (raw)

Purchase unsalted nuts and seeds, which may be found at many natural grocery and health food stores. Raw nuts rather than roasted ones have been shown to have more nutritional properties, but they can be more difficult for some people to digest. If you have such a sensitivity, soak raw nuts before consuming them whole or using them in nut butters and desserts. Soak almonds for eight hours, walnuts for four hours, and cashews for two hours. Allow nuts to dry thoroughly before use or use a dehydrator to speed up the process.

Like walnuts and walnut oils, chia and flaxseeds have high levels of omega-3 fatty acids and serve as great supplements to seafood and fish.

Natural Sweeteners

There have been various debates over which natural sweeteners are considered Paleo. Some new research suggests that all sweeteners, from honey to sugar, have the same effect on the body, so some Paleo purists try to reduce all sweeteners, regardless. Others choose raw honey, raw agave nectar, grade B pure maple syrup, and dates over refined sugars because some studies suggest they have less impact on insulin levels and contain trace amounts of antioxidants and minerals.

Some Paleo eaters use coconut sugar or crystals in baking because they have a low-glycemic index and work like regular sugar. Others consider molasses acceptable for Paleo because it is less refined and contains some minerals and nutrients. Dates are an even better choice. They are naturally sweet and great for baking because of their consistency when pureed. As with sweet potatoes and fruits, consume these sweeteners in moderation.

Herbs and Spices

Keeping a variety of fresh herbs and spices on hand will spruce up meals without the need for extra salt. Certain herbs have been shown to have nutritional properties. For example, ginger has been shown to aid in digestion, while garlic and parsley have strong anti-inflammatory and antioxidant benefits. Herbs should be stored in the refrigerator like flowers—place the herb stems upright in a glass with cool water. Ginger may be peeled, cut up into smaller pieces, and frozen for last-minute needs.

Condiments

Certain condiments like vinegars, mustards, and hot sauce may fit into the Paleo lifestyle and are a great way to add flavor to your food. However, it's important to read labels carefully and avoid brands with added sodium, sugars, and stabilizers like guar gum as well as preservatives and additives you can't pronounce.

Beverages

By far, water is the best beverage when following the Paleo lifestyle. Aim for at least eight glasses a day. Some people drink far more than this amount to flush toxins from their body and ensure ample hydration.

Squeezing a little fresh lemon and/or lime juice in your water may make it more palatable. Though lemon and lime juices taste acidic, they actually have the opposite effect on the body, improving alkaline levels, which can help reduce inflammation.

Other Paleo-friendly beverages include:

- **Carbonated water with a squeeze of lemon or lime:** Drink this in moderation, however, because too much bubbly may cause digestive issues and bloating for some people.
- **Coffee:** Some Paleo purists avoid caffeine, but others allow small amounts, which can improve workouts and mental clarity.
- **Tea:** Choose from green, black, oolong, and herbal teas, again in moderation to monitor caffeine levels.
- **Unsweetened coconut water:** This is naturally low in sugar. It's also high in potassium, which can prevent muscle cramping and aid in hydration. Make sure to read labels carefully and choose brands without added sugars.
- Unsweetened nut milks

Supplements

Many Paleo eaters incorporate supplements to further enhance nutritional absorption and stabilize hormone levels. Taking a multivitamin can fill in nutrition gaps, but taking certain vitamins individually can have even stronger health benefits.

- Calcium strengthens bones.
- Fish oil (mercury-free) repairs muscles, boosts brain activity, improves emotional health, "greases" joints, clears skin, and strengthens hair, eyes, and nails.
- Probiotics aid in digestion and removing toxins from the body. Taking a probiotic supplement is more effective than consuming yogurt with live cultures, which would require consuming large amounts of yogurt for the same health benefits.
- Vitamin B boosts metabolism and energy levels.
- Vitamin C helps repair muscles and boost immunity.
- Vitamin D strengthens the immune system's ability to ward off illness, especially when the supplement is combined with the sunlight's natural source of vitamin D.

FOODS TO AVOID

Grains

Though Paleo is not officially labeled as a "gluten-free" way of eating, the same idea applies. Many people walk around wondering why they suffer from digestive problems and everyday bloating, only to find when they eliminate wheat, gluten—and in the case of Paleo—other grains from their diet, these problems clear up.

According to Paleo nutritionists and other scientists, grains—even "whole-wheat" kinds and oats—are heavily processed foods that can have adverse effects on the body. In addition to digestion issues, some suggest that too many grains can lead to chronic inflammation in the body, and they don't burn as efficiently as protein and fats, which can lead to increased body fat production and stubborn, excess fat storage over the long term.

Here is a list of grains and starches to avoid:

- Amaranth
- Barley
- Bread
- Buckwheat
- Corn and cornmeal
- Kamut
- Millet
- Oats
- Rice: brown and white
- Spelt
- Tapioca
- Wheat
- White potatoes

Legumes

Paleo nutritionists and other researchers point to legumes—including beans, soy, and peanuts—as contributors to "leaky gut" syndrome, which can cause digestion problems and potentially lead to autoimmune diseases and issues.

Here is a list of legumes to avoid:

- Beans, including dried and canned
- Peanuts and peanut butter
- Peas
- Soy

Sugar and Artificial Sweeteners

There is no shortage of research showing the damages that refined sugars may cause. These sugars—in the form of granulated sugar and high-fructose corn syrup found in many baked goods, processed foods, and sugary sodas—raise insulin levels instantly when ingested. Large doses over time may cause chronic problems with insulin production and resistance, leading to prediabetic and diabetic conditions.

Furthermore, sugar makes you hungrier. Refined sugars do not burn as efficiently as other wholesome foods, and they can stimulate the appetite hormone leptin, even when your body does not require food.

Research shows that even artificial sweeteners—including those claiming to be "natural," such as those made from the stevia plant—can raise blood sugar levels by tricking your body into thinking you've eaten sugar.

Here is a list of sugary foods, refined sugars, and artificial sweeteners to avoid:

- Aspartame
- Brown rice syrup
- Candy
- Cane syrup
- Chocolate: white, milk, and some dark
- Corn syrup and high-fructose corn syrup
- Saccharine
- Splenda
- Stevia
- Sugar: white, brown, and sugar in the raw
- Sugar alcohols: maltitol and sorbitol
- Sucralose

Dairy

Though the latest U.S. Department of Agriculture (USDA) guidelines push dairy as part of a complete diet, many researchers believe that cow's milk can actually cause more harm than good to the body and that it's not needed for good nutritional health.

While many people suffer from lactose intolerance, the high levels of lactic acid and presence of casein, a dairy protein, in milk can cause indigestion problems for people even without a formal diagnosis. Moreover, the added acidity in cow's milk can also contribute to chronic inflammation.

Some research suggests that adults, and even children, do not need to drink any milk once weaned from human breast milk, and that cow's milk may prevent adequate calcium and other nutritional absorption. Get your calcium from other edible sources, such as nut milks and dark, leafy greens.

Some cow's milk runs the risk of containing hormones added to livestock feed. Ingesting these hormones can throw your hormone levels out of balance and lead to a host of other problems, including weight gain. Many cheeses contain excess levels of salt compared to "cleaner" sources of protein.

Some Paleo followers eat small amounts of cultured and grass-fed butter and sheep's milk or goat's milk yogurts, because they don't contain as much lactose as cow's milk, causing fewer digestive problems. Those foods are not included in *The Paleo Beginners Guide*, but if you do choose to incorporate them, consume them in moderation (no more than one serving a day and no more than three servings per week).

Deli Meats

Deli meats, including turkey, roast beef, pastrami, ham, and some bacon, should be avoided, because they often contain too much sodium as well as added nitrates and preservatives.

Roast your own turkey and beef to avoid high sodium levels and preservatives and additives. Thinly slice and refrigerate the meat for quick lunches and snacks.

Additives and Preservatives

Many processed foods, and even some proteins and processed meats, contain a long list of artificial colorings and dyes, stabilizers, and other chemical additives for flavor and longer shelf life. Studies suggest additives and preservatives introduce harmful acids that can cause inflammation in the body, and others such as lecithin might be safe but they're made from "cheap" ingredients like soybeans, which are highly processed by themselves. Carrageenan, for example, a thickener found in some non-dairy alternatives like coconut milk, coconut yogurt, and processed meats, does not sound harmful but has been shown to add to "leaky gut" syndrome, when the intestinal walls develop holes that allow toxins from the waste stream to flood back into the body. The Paleo lifestyle discourages the consumptions of all food additives for a "cleaner," fresher diet closer to what our ancestors might have eaten.

Sodium

Salt is limited in the Paleo lifestyle because of the avoidance of processed foods. Table salt—often enhanced with iodine—contains higher concentrations of sodium than other more natural, less processed salts because of the smaller grains.

Some recipes in the book call for sea salt. When selecting sea salt, look for Himalayan pink sea salt or Celtic sea salt, which contain healthful minerals and are less refined. Some *fleur de sel* and gray sea salts also contain traces of good minerals.

If you buy broth and tomatoes, carefully read the labels on those that claim to have less sodium. Sometimes even so-called low-sodium broths can have more than the recommended daily amount. As a result, pickles, olives, and other canned goods are not in the Paleo diet.

Starchy Vegetables and Fruits

Starchy vegetables can raise insulin levels just like sugar does, and they don't burn fat as efficiently as their more fiber-rich siblings. Starchy fruits and vegetables to avoid include:

- Bananas
- White potatoes: baking, russet, and Yukon gold

Some Paleo followers eat bananas in small amounts, but they are excluded from this book. Test out your response to bananas by incorporating a little bit into a smoothie or eating half of one with some almond butter and listen to your body. If you feel even hungrier or experience a "sugar rush" feeling, it could indicate a spike in blood sugar.

Canned Fruits, Fruit Juices, and Sodas

Some fruits have more sugar than others, especially those canned or jarred in syrup with other sugars added. Fruit juices, because they do not have any of the beneficial fiber that whole fruits do, can cause blood sugar spikes.

Of course, sugary sodas and other sugar-laden beverages (even some ice tea brands) should be avoided because they introduce excess amounts of sugars and calories without any nutritional benefits.

Alcohol

Paleo purists tend to avoid alcohol, but if you do choose to imbibe, some are better than others.

Avoid beer because of the use of grains in production, and stay clear of dark-colored spirits like rum, whiskey, and scotch, which tend to have more sugars and can spike blood sugar. Watch out for liqueurs and cream-based spirits as well.

Some say tequila and mescal have less effect on blood sugar. Wine is considered less harmful than hard alcohols, but it should be consumed in moderation. Red wine contains more antioxidants than white, making it a better choice.

PALEO FAQS

I'm vegetarian. Can I still follow the Paleo lifestyle?

While it is possible to eat vegetarian on the Paleo lifestyle, it may be difficult, as many meals contain meat and seafood as the main sources of protein. While legumes and grains are discouraged, nuts and seeds contain good amounts of protein as well as eggs. Pescatarians are still able to enjoy the omega-3 and protein benefits of fish. Vegetarians may also choose grass-fed whey or hemp seed powder for additional protein sources. Some manufacturers make amino acid powder blends that combine with water or coconut water for an additional protein source, but be careful to look for added sugars.

Most Paleo purists avoid soy because it is a legume. That includes tofu, tempeh, and other soy-based products. Others eat some tofu, as long as it is minimally processed, or better yet, sprouted for easier digestion. Eating too much soy has been shown to throw hormones out of balance, which can have adverse effects on weight loss efforts and long-term health, especially in men.

How can I ensure I am getting enough fiber in my diet if I am omitting grains?

When it comes to fiber, even whole grains can't compete with fresh fruits and vegetables. While many grain products are enriched with vitamin B, there are more natural, better ways of getting this important nutrient, particularly by eating quality meats and eggs. Taking a supplement can also provide three times the amount of vitamin B compared to eating a shopping cart load of baked goods. If you're concerned about fiber intake, try adding a fiber supplement to your diet.

Some research says saturated fat from meat is bad for you. How can Paleo be considered healthful?

The Paleo lifestyle encourages choosing pasture-raised meats rather than commodity meat from animals raised in feedlots and treated with hormones and/or daily antibiotics. Animals raised on mainly grass diets have higher levels of heart-healthful omega-3 fatty acids and less saturated fat than commercial meat. Avoidance of dairy also helps limit excess saturated fat intake.

Do I have to exercise?

Yes! Exercise, especially strength training, in conjunction with a healthful diet, will speed up fat loss and build muscle. If you are new to exercise, start slowly. If you spend most of your time at the gym spinning, running, or going like a hamster on an elliptical machine, add some strength training to your routine. Or take some classes that offer high-intensity interval workouts to bump up your fat-burning capabilities.

Why can't I eat beans?

Many beans, even dried beans, are heavily processed and grown in less than ideal conditions.

How is Paleo different than a gluten-free diet?

While Paleo encourages avoiding gluten in the form of whole wheat, wheat products, and processed foods with added gluten, this way of eating also discourages other "gluten-free" grains like corn and amaranth, which can cause issues with chronic inflammation. Quinoa, touted for its health benefits as of late, may be confusing for Paleo purists. Though it is a seed, it contains saponins, which can form holes in intestinal membranes and contribute to "leaky gut," a condition in which toxins from the digestive path leak back out into the blood and body, causing inflammation.

Why do some of the recipes call for boxed broths and tomatoes?

Many canned products are made with bisphenol A, also known as BPA, which is a carbon-based chemical used in packaging. Experts have said BPA from aluminum and plastic packaging can potentially leach into foods. Considered carcinogens, BPAs have been linked to certain cancer risks and can introduce harmful toxins in the body. As always, when selecting products packaged in cartons, make sure they don't contain additives or preservatives.

Will I get enough calcium in my diet since I'm not eating dairy?

Not eating dairy may even increase your calcium levels. Since cow's milk is high in acid, it can block the absorption of calcium. Many nut milks contain ample amounts of calcium (make sure to shake these products thoroughly before using). Dark, leafy greens, like kale and spinach, are another great source of calcium. If you're concerned about calcium intake outside of food sources, consider taking a supplement as well as extra vitamin D, and try to get ten minutes of natural light or artificial sunlight (using a light box) a day.

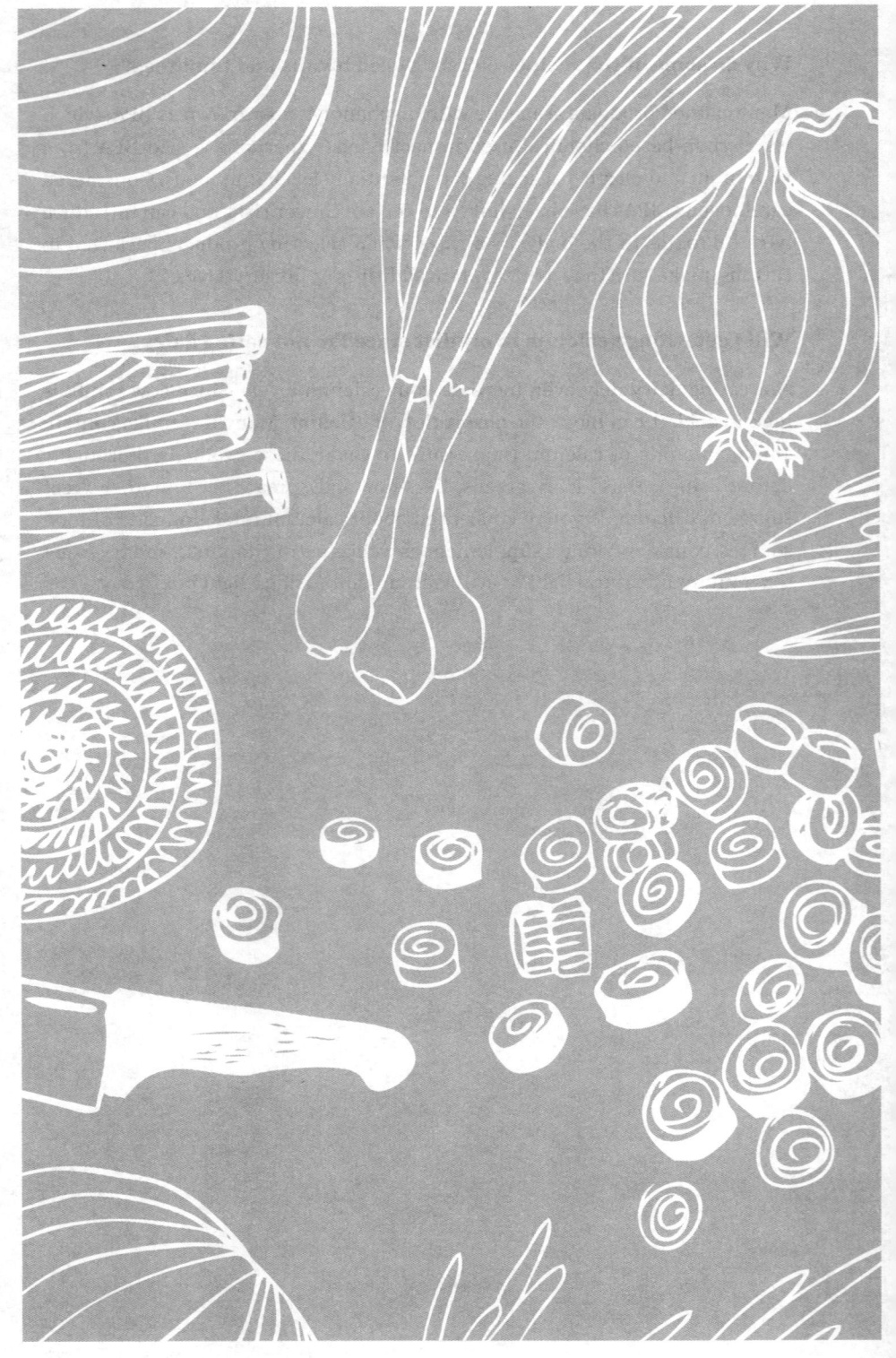

CHAPTER TWO

How to Use the Paleo Diet Meal Plan

Boredom. It's the main reason many people don't stick with diets. Eating the same thing, day in and day out, is an easy way to succumb to unhealthful cravings and set yourself up for failure.

The Paleo lifestyle is about variety and fresher, cleaner, better-tasting food that will literally change what you crave. Sugar and salt junkies who go the Paleo route often find the foods they once ate as too sweet, too salty, and not nearly as delicious as the new, wholesome meals.

Still, adopting a Paleo lifestyle doesn't mean you can flip a switch and reap all the benefits at once. That's why, by following a set meal plan, you can familiarize yourself and get comfortable with the new foods and slowly flush out the cravings for less healthful options. Meal plans, such as the one in this book, take the guesswork out of a new way of eating and help you stay focused, organized, and inspired.

By having a clear food "map," you can rest assured that each meal will be unique. Having a clearly laid-out shopping list will help you cut down on wasted time and money. And with a slew of exciting and easy-to-follow recipes at your fingertips, you'll be able to spend the next month cooking with ease and enjoyment.

MAKE THE MOST OF YOUR MEAL PLAN

While meal plans mean prescribed breakfasts, lunches, and dinners, know that after following the planned twenty-eight days, the options for continuing your Paleo lifestyle are endless. Eating the Paleo way at its simplest means combining healthful proteins with vegetables and a little healthful fat in their purest, most wholesome form.

Before heading out to stock your pantry and refrigerator, make sure you're up to speed on the Paleo food groups, knowing that there are far more foods to enjoy than to avoid. Clear out your cupboards, refrigerator, and freezer to make room for cleaner, energy-boosting foods. Give yourself a little extra time on your first grocery run so you can choose produce wisely, read labels, and ask your butcher questions, if necessary. Remember to shop, cook, and freeze in bulk, especially proteins, berries, and nuts, so you'll always have ingredients on hand for quick meals and a wide range of options. If anything, shopping this way will excite your creativity during and well beyond this twenty-eight-day plan.

Once you're comfortable with the recipes and guidelines in *The Paleo Beginners Guide*, create your own dishes using a combination of proteins, produce, and fats to try new flavors and pairings.

LEARN TO READ FOOD LABELS

These days, deciphering food labels at the grocery store may be tricky and time-consuming. Claims like "all natural" and "hormone-free" don't always mean what they say. For example, by law all poultry must be raised without hormones, so calling chicken "hormone-free" is a moot point. Even "free-range" does not mean the same thing as "pastured," which is more ideal because it means the animal ate only grass throughout its life. Sadly, many of these labels are simply marketing tactics food manufacturers use to entice customers to buy their products.

Some Paleo purists avoid chicken, pork, and beef sausages altogether, while others make an exception if they contain only natural ingredients. When reading labels, look for yourself, and if there are ingredients you can't pronounce or noticeable preservatives on a product, move on to another one. And watch the sodium content in foods like these as well as in broths, crushed tomatoes, and nut butters. Even those labeled "low sodium" may still contain higher levels than unsalted versions or sauces, stocks, and condiments you could make yourself.

Reading Food Labels

The Paleo eating plan focuses on fresh vegetables, fruits, and proteins, which you buy raw and prepare yourself. But anytime you buy packaged food—even items labeled "natural," "organic," "nonfat," "low-sodium," "no sugar added," and the like—it's crucial to read the ingredients list and the Nutrition Facts label. Unless you do, you have no way of knowing exactly what's in your food.

Inspect the ingredients list and reject any food that contains refined grains, excess sugar or salt, or anything on the "Foods to Avoid" list in Chapter One. Then look at the size of the print on the ingredients label. If it's too small to read, that's a clue that there might be a whole lot of ingredients in the product. More ingredients often means more stuff that's bad for you, such as artificial flavors, sweeteners, and colors, or a whole laboratory's worth of emulsifiers, flavor enhancers (such as monosodium glutamate), preservatives, stabilizers, and thickeners. Some of the mystery matter might include hidden sugars, high-fructose corn syrup, bad fats, or sodium. If you see a lot of ingredients that you can't pronounce or decipher, it's a good idea to put the package back on the shelf.

The government-mandated Nutrition Facts label, that information box printed on every packaged food product in the store, is a treasure trove of Paleo data. It doesn't tell you everything you'd like to know, but it's still a valuable tool. Take a look at the example here.

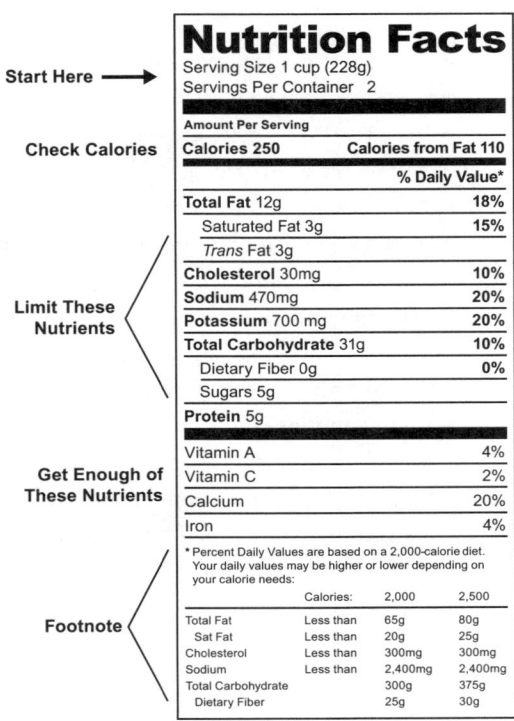

The "serving size" and "servings per container" at the top of the label give you an understanding of how much food is actually in the package. The "calories" line indicates how many calories and fat-based calories are in *one* serving (based on the stated serving size). Below that, the lines for nutrients, from "total fat" down to "protein," give the weight (in grams) of each nutrient that's contained in a single serving.

Another measurement, the "percent daily value," is given for each of the nutrients as well as for some vitamins and minerals. Percent daily value is based on government recommendations for how much of a given substance a 2,000-calorie-per-day diet should include. For instance, the 15 percent figure for saturated fat in the example label means one serving contains 15 percent of the saturated fat you should eat in a 2,000-calorie day. If a vitamin or mineral doesn't appear in the Nutrition Facts label, the food isn't a significant source of the nutrient. The basic rule is that a food is considered low in any nutrients with a daily value of 5 percent or less, and high in those with a daily value of 20 percent or more.

SHOPPING TIPS

The Paleo lifestyle means eating wholesome, unprocessed foods, so shop the perimeter of the grocery store or supermarket. There, you'll find most of the produce and meat offerings. The inner aisles are reserved mainly for boxed and packaged foods, which you won't need, except perhaps for crushed and diced tomatoes, broths, oils, nuts, some condiments, Paleo baking needs, and non-dairy beverages like canned coconut milk, typically found in the ethnic food aisles. Other non-dairy beverages, namely almond milk, may be found near dairy products in the refrigerated sections.

When purchasing Paleo-friendly packaged foods, again, read the labels carefully. Make sure there are no added sugars, preservatives, stabilizers, or other ingredients you can't pronounce, and always check the sodium content. Unsalted, roasted, or raw nuts and nut butters are best, while no-salt-added tomatoes and broth can be helpful for quick soups and sauces. Choose tomatoes packaged in cartons rather than canned ones to avoid potential BPAs or carbon-based chemicals used in plastic and aluminum packaging. Some research has pointed to BPAs as carcinogens that can elevate the risk of cancer.

STOCK YOUR PANTRY

The first step in stocking your pantry for the Paleo lifestyle is to discard all non-Paleo packaged goods, such as bread, rice, pasta, cookies, crackers, artificial sweeteners, and any grains as well as canned soups and beans. By removing these from the get-go, you also remove temptation from the house. To avoid waste, donate unopened goods to a local food drive.

Take a look at your freezer. Toss out any ice cream, waffles, and bagels as well as other frozen breads, dairy, and sugar-laden products. Remove starchy, non-Paleo vegetables like frozen peas and potatoes.

Discard any juices, sodas (except for seltzer water or club soda), yogurt, and non-Paleo condiments like sugary ketchup and soy, teriyaki, and hoisin sauce from the refrigerator.

Now it's time to go shopping. While many of these items are listed in your weekly meal plan shopping lists, here is a complete list of Paleo-approved pantry items to keep on hand for your new way of eating.

Oils

Refrigerate nut oils to prevent them from going rancid.

- Almond
- Avocado
- Cold-pressed, extra-virgin olive
- Coconut
- Flaxseed (unfiltered)
- Grape-seed (optional)
- Hazelnut
- Walnut

Other Fats

These ingredients are not used in this book, but some Paleo followers choose to have them on hand for cooking and baking.

- Butter made from pastured cow's milk
- Palm shortening

Nuts and Seeds

Refrigerate or freeze nuts and seeds to prevent them from going rancid.

- Almonds (raw, roasted and unsalted)
- Brazil nuts (raw)
- Chia seeds

- Flaxseeds
- Hazelnuts (raw, roasted and unsalted)
- Macadamia nuts (raw, roasted and unsalted)
- Pistachios (raw, roasted and unsalted)
- Pumpkin seeds
- Sesame seeds
- Sunflower seeds
- Walnuts (raw)

Nut Butters

- Almond (unsalted and raw or roasted)
- Cashew (unsalted and raw or roasted)
- Sunflower (unsalted and roasted)

Baking Items

Store coconut and nut flours in the freezer to prevent them from going rancid.

- Almond meal and almond flour
- Baking powder
- Baking soda
- Cacao powder, raw
- Chocolate, unsweetened
- Cocoa, unsweetened
- Coconut flakes, unsweetened
- Coconut flour
- Vanilla extract, pure

Natural Sweeteners

- Agave nectar, raw
- Honey, raw
- Maple syrup, grade B, pure
- Medjool dates

Vinegars

- Apple cider
- Balsamic and aged balsamic
- Coconut
- Red wine

Condiments

- Dijon mustard
- Horseradish root
- Hot sauce (no sugar added)
- Salsa (no sugar or preservatives added)

Other Pantry Items

- Broth, low-sodium vegetable and chicken, in cartons (preferably organic)
- Dried fruits, unsweetened (cranberries, blueberries, cherries, goji berries)
- Maca powder
- Nori seaweed sheets
- Red peppers, jarred, roasted
- Soy sauce, gluten-free, low sodium (tamari, Bragg Liquid Aminos)
- Tomatoes, no salt added, boxed

Seasonings and Spices

- Allspice
- Bay leaves
- Black peppercorns
- Cayenne pepper
- Cinnamon
- Coriander
- Cumin
- Fennel seed
- Garlic powder
- Onion powder
- Oregano
- Red pepper flakes
- Sea salt (Himalayan, Celtic)
- Tarragon
- Thyme

BASIC EQUIPMENT AND SUPPLIES

The following is a list of suggested equipment and supplies you'll need when following the Paleo lifestyle:

Very Important

- Blender, food processor, and/or handheld blender
- BPA-free and/or glass containers for leftovers meals and snacks
- Cutting board
- Freezer-safe plastic bags
- Jars for storing salsas, sauces, dressings, and other homemade condiments
- Large roasting pan for chicken, turkeys, and roasts
- Liquid measuring containers
- Measuring cups and spoons
- Meat thermometer
- Mixing bowls
- Oven-safe sheet trays, baking pans, and glass baking dishes for roasting and casseroles
- Parchment paper or aluminum foil
- Pepper grinder
- Rubber spatulas and tongs
- Sharp knives
- Stainless steel or ceramic sauté pans and pots (be leery of non-stick pans and pots, which can leach toxic chemicals into foods if damaged or scratched)

Somewhat Important

- Dutch oven or other large ovenproof dish
- Large stockpot
- Mesh or vegetable-saver bags for extending produce freshness
- Microwave-safe bowls and containers
- Muffin pans and bread pans
- Salad spinner

Useful But Not as Important

- Dehydrator for homemade jerky, dried fruits, and drying soaked nuts
- Microwave egg cooker
- Slow cooker
- Smoothie shaker
- Spice (or coffee) grinder
- Spiralizer to make noodle-like strands out of cucumbers, zucchini, and carrots

MAKE THE PALEO DIET WORK FOR YOU

Following the Paleo diet will revive and revitalize you. You'll have newfound energy and lose weight. An important part of eating Paleo, however, means preparing many of your own meals and snacks. Here are some tips to improve your shopping, cooking, and food-saving techniques to make the most of your money, time, and resources. By following these tips, you'll soon improve your health and well-being with Paleo's clean and fresh way of eating.

- **Buy in bulk and freeze extra meat.** For instance, if buying ground beef for burgers, buy a little more for tacos or chili that week. Remember to use the entire portion once thawed; refreezing thawed meat can introduce harmful bacteria. Wrap burger patties and chicken breasts individually before freezing, so you can take out the correct portion sizes.
- **Cook in bulk.** When making chili, for example, double the recipe and freeze the extra chili in individual portions for quick lunches or dinners. When cooking fish, flake the leftovers and form them into "burgers" for a quick lunch the next day. If you find yourself with extra vegetables at the end of the week, steam and add them to salads.
- **Experiment with different poultry, meat, and seafood.** The called-for meat in most of the recipes throughout this book may easily be substituted with something else. Use ground beef or bison in place of ground turkey or chicken, or chicken breasts instead of steak. Do pay attention to cooking times, as they will differ.

- **Keep healthful snacks on hand.** Maintain a variety of healthful snacks for when hunger strikes. See the Appendix for Paleo-approved snacks.
- **Eat vegetables at every meal.** Add fresh spinach to soups and smoothies, mix bell peppers and carrots into meatloaf and chili, and create imaginative salads.
- **Enjoy fruit in moderation.** Eat Paleo-approved, low-sugar fruit earlier in the day to keep blood sugar stable.
- **Stock up on homemade or Paleo-friendly staples.** Pestos, salsas, salad dressings, oils, fresh herbs, and dried spices will add layers of flavor to your dishes.
- **Eat a healthful fat at each meal.** Top salads and soups with nuts and seeds for crunch or slices of avocado for richness. Add a tablespoon of nut butter to smoothies, and use good-quality oils when preparing meat and vegetables.
- **Subscribe to a community-supported agriculture (CSA) share.** This will help you source fresh, sustainably produced vegetables, fruit, meat, and eggs directly from local farmers and at more competitive prices than farmers' markets.
- **Freeze extra berries.** Spread berries on a baking sheet in a single layer and freeze them until firm. Transfer the frozen berries to a bag and store them in the freezer for smoothies.
- **Save your diced veggies.** Freeze extra onion, bell peppers, and zucchini for cooked dishes like soups and chili, but note that vegetables are softer and release more water when thawed.
- **Refrigerate or freeze nuts.** Nuts tend to go rancid even when stored in cool, dark cupboards. They will last longer when stored in the freezer. Some nut oils like walnut, almond, and hazelnut oil should be kept in the refrigerator to prevent rancidity.
- **Make exercise a priority.** Following the Paleo lifestyle means eating well, but it also means moving more for both weight loss and mental health. Many Paleo eaters focus on high-intensity workouts and movements as well as an equal balance of strength training and cardio to build muscle, burn fat, combat stress, and boost energy levels.

DINING OUT

Those who follow a Paleo lifestyle have no problem dining out in restaurants. With the exception of pizzerias and some fast-food chains, restaurants everywhere can prepare dishes to your liking. By scanning the menu carefully and making some simple decisions and substitutions, if necessary, there are plenty of choices when eating out.

- **Go for the protein.** Look for meat- or fish-based entrées and appetizers first. Choose sautéed, steamed, or roasted vegetables or salads as sides over starchier ones like fries, potatoes, grains, and rice.
- **Avoid fried foods.** Most fried foods are breaded and cooked in unhealthful fats, such as palm oil. Look closely at appetizer menus, where the bulk of fried items exist. Order a salad, oysters, or a shrimp cocktail instead.
- **Skip the bread basket.** Kindly ask your server to remove the basket or politely decline when offered. Out of sight is out of mind.
- **Read between the lines.** At Italian restaurants, watch out for dishes labeled "Milanese," which means breaded, or "Parmesan," which indicates layered with cheese. Many sauces and dressings labeled as "creamy" are made with dairy products as well as flour, cornstarch, or other thickeners.
- **Carefully examine dressings.** Skip ranch and blue cheese dressings, which contain diary. Opt for balsamic, Italian, and other vinaigrettes, but only if they are made in-house. Many packaged dressings contain hidden sugars, sodium, and other preservatives. In a pinch, a squeeze of lemon can brighten any salad, or ask for oil and vinegar to create your own vinaigrette.
- **Modify your salad.** Salads are a Paleo-friendly choice, but ask your server to omit fried wontons, croutons, rice noodles, dried fruits (most restaurant versions will be made with sugar), and cheeses.
- **Choose alcohol wisely, or skip it.** While most Paleo plans discourage alcohol consumption, wine and champagne in small amounts are acceptable in some circles. Avoid beer and spirits like whisky, bourbon, and rum, which contain more sugar and carbohydrates than spirits like vodka and gin. Even better, some say agave-based tequila and mescal have less effect on blood sugar, but skip the sugary margarita and ask for a mix with sparkling water and lime instead.

- **Make your own soda.** Instead of regular or diet sodas, which contain artificial sweeteners and other non-Paleo additives, ask for seltzer or sparkling water with lemon or lime wedges for a healthier alternative. Note that club soda seltzer does contain small amounts of added sodium, so consume these moderately if seltzer or sparkling water is not available.
- **Build a better burger.** When ordering a burger, ask for more lettuce and tomatoes in place of a bun.
- **Make Mexican Paleo.** Most Mexican restaurants fit into a Paleo lifestyle. Look for meat- or fish-based entrées, such as fajitas or fish tacos, but hold the tortillas. Of course, guacamole, fresh lime wedges, and cilantro make for great toppers to any dish.

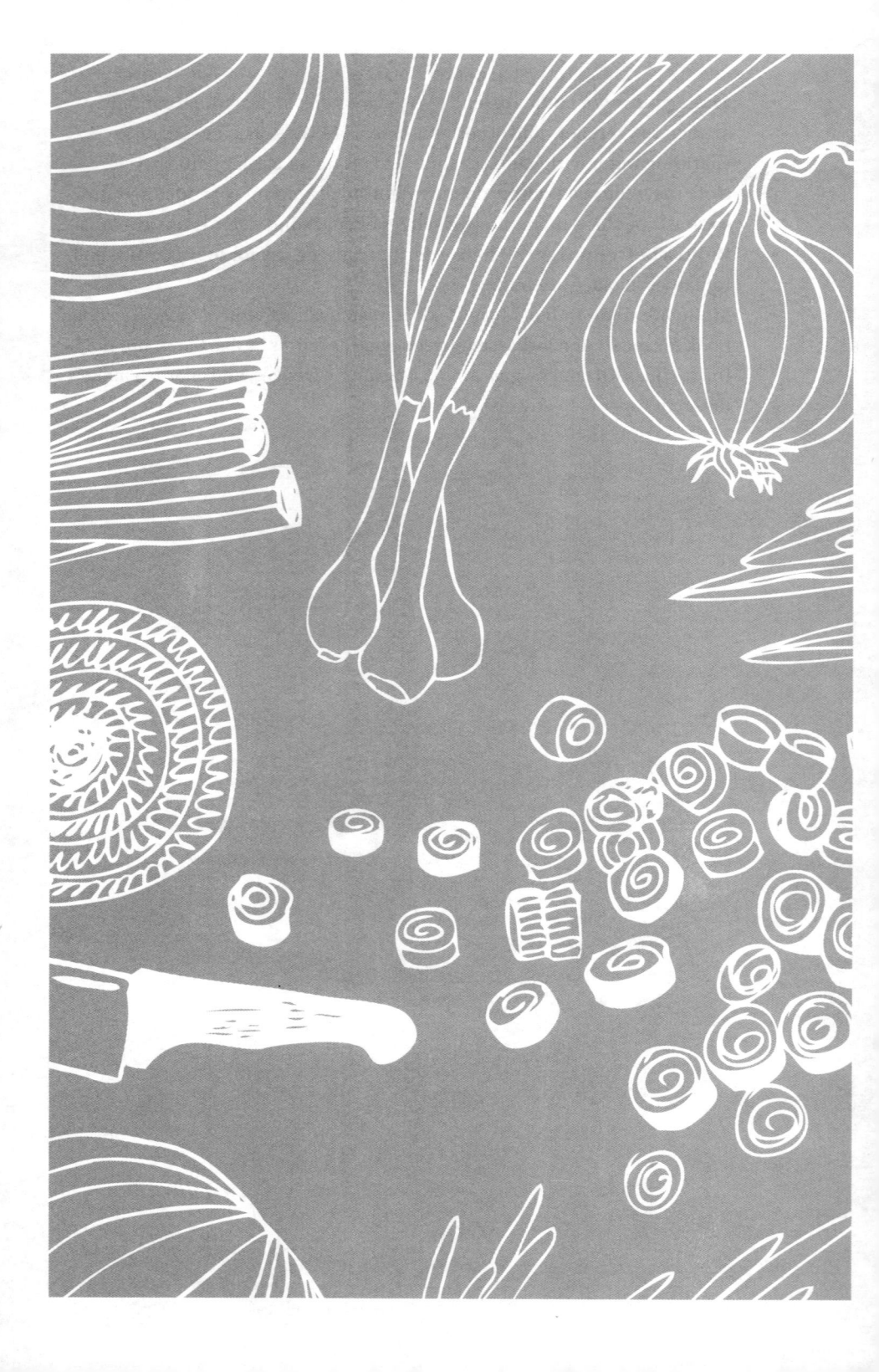

PART TWO

Putting the Paleo Diet Meal Plan into Action

CHAPTER THREE WEEK ONE

CHAPTER FOUR WEEK TWO

CHAPTER FIVE WEEK THREE

The following twenty-eight-day meal plan will give you the inspiration, guidance, and enthusiasm you need to begin your new Paleo life. This section is broken down into four chapters, one for each week. Each week includes a seven-day meal plan with four meals for each day—breakfast, lunch, dinner, and dessert—as well as a recipe for each meal. To keep hunger in check, enjoy one or two snacks from the suggestions in the Appendix.

Handy, detailed shopping lists help you purchase the right Paleo-friendly ingredients, while preparation tips offer time-saving ideas. Daily tips will give you a little dose of encouragement and inspiration. Prepare the homemade sauces and staples in Chapter Ten, so you'll have flavorful condiments readily available. If you're pressed for time at lunch, prepare parts of the midday recipes ahead of time, or move cooking-intensive lunches to dinnertime and eat a salad instead.

CHAPTER THREE

Week One

WEEK ONE MEAL PLAN

Day One

Breakfast
Frittata with Bacon, Collard Greens, and Scallions
Lunch
Smoked Salmon Sushi Roll-Ups
Dinner
Korean Barbecue Beef Lettuce Wraps
Dessert
Almond Butter Bites

> **Daily Tip:** Don't be too concerned with counting calories, but do make an effort to keep your portion sizes appropriate.

Day Two

Breakfast
Lox, Eggs, and Onion Scramble
Lunch
Chile-Rubbed Chicken Fajitas with Avocados
Dinner
Cuban Pulled Pork
Dessert
Chia Seed Pudding

Daily Tip: Eat without distractions. Before you sit down to a meal, turn off the TV, tablets, and smartphones. Save books and magazines for another time. Enjoy and savor each bite to feel fully satisfied.

Day Three

Breakfast
Blueberry Power Breakfast Smoothie
Lunch
Leftover frittata from breakfast on Day 1 and a small green salad with 1 tablespoon each of Paleo-approved oil and vinegar
Dinner
Chicken Vesuvio with Sweet Potatoes
Dessert
Chocolate-Strawberry "Milk" Shake

Daily Tip: Don't be afraid to use leftovers! Use leftover cooked meats in salads and soups or pair them with vegetables for a quick meal.

Day Four

Breakfast
Maple-Fennel Breakfast Sausage with Scrambled Eggs
Lunch
Pulled pork from dinner on Day 2 on a bed of greens
Dinner
Halibut Steaks with Salsa Verde
Dessert
Blueberry Macadamia Squares

Daily Tip: Drink plenty of water. Add a lime or lemon wedge, a few cucumber slices, or some fresh mint leaves to your water glass or bottle for a little flavor variety.

Day Five

Breakfast
Nutty Fruit Bars

Lunch
Waldorf Salad with Chicken, Apples, and Walnuts made with chicken leftover from dinner on Day 3

Dinner
Herbed Turkey Meatballs with Spaghetti Squash

Dessert
Chocolate Coconut Truffles

> **Daily Tip:** Save and freeze the bones and carcasses from chicken and turkey recipes to make broths and soups.

Day Six

Breakfast
Poached Eggs with Spicy Tomato Sauce

Lunch
Chicken "Noodle" Soup using Chicken Broth (page 158)

Dinner
Chard-Wrapped Arctic Char with Balsamic Glaze

Dessert
Coconut Date "Blondies"

> **Daily Tip:** Slow down and enjoy your meals. If you eat too quickly, you may end up with a false sense of hunger once you've eaten your portioned-out meal.

Day Seven

Breakfast
Blueberry-Almond Paleo Pancakes
Lunch
Curried Egg Salad
Dinner
Standing Rib Roast with Mustard-Horseradish Sauce
Dessert
Quick and Easy Microwave Brownie

> **Daily Tip:** Use an all-natural produce wash to clean fruits and vegetables as soon as you get home from the market or grocery store so they're ready when you need them. Apples, cucumbers, and bell peppers in particular are often sprayed with waxes, even the organic versions.

WEEK ONE RECIPES

Breakfast

- Frittata with Bacon, Collard Greens, and Scallions
- Lox, Eggs, and Onion Scramble
- Blueberry Power Breakfast Smoothie
- Maple-Fennel Breakfast Sausage with Scrambled Eggs
- Nutty Fruit Bars
- Poached Eggs with Spicy Tomato Sauce
- Blueberry-Almond Paleo Pancakes

Lunch

- Smoked Salmon Sushi Roll-Ups
- Chile-Rubbed Chicken Fajitas with Avocados
- Waldorf Salad with Chicken, Apples, and Walnuts
- Chicken "Noodle" Soup
- Curried Egg Salad

Dinner

- Korean Barbecue Beef Lettuce Wraps
- Cuban Pulled Pork
- Chicken Vesuvio with Sweet Potatoes
- Halibut Steaks with Salsa Verde
- Herbed Turkey Meatballs with Spaghetti Squash
- Chard-Wrapped Arctic Char with Balsamic Glaze
- Standing Rib Roast with Mustard-Horseradish Sauce

Dessert

- Almond Butter Bites
- Chia Seed Pudding
- Chocolate-Strawberry "Milk" Shake
- Blueberry Macadamia Squares
- Chocolate Coconut Truffles
- Coconut Date "Blondies"
- Quick and Easy Microwave Brownie

WEEK ONE SHOPPING LIST

To prepare your meals for this week, stock your pantry for future weeks, and prepare the recipes in Chapter Ten, purchase the following items:

Pantry Items

Note: This is a full list of Paleo-approved pantry, baking, and refrigerated items to have on hand for the next thirty days. Refer back to this complete list when reviewing shopping lists for weeks two, three, and four.

- Agave nectar
- Apple cider vinegar
- Avocado oil
- Baking powder
- Baking soda
- Broth, no salt added, vegetable and/or chicken
- Cherries, dried, unsweetened
- Cacao paste, raw
- Cacao powder, raw
- Cocoa powder, unsweetened
- Coconut oil
- Coconut water, unsweetened
- Cranberries, cherries, or blueberries, dried, unsweetened
- Dates, Medjool, pitted

- Dijon mustard
- Grape-seed oil
- Honey, raw
- Maca powder (optional)
- Maple syrup, grade B, pure
- Nori sheets
- Olive oil, extra-virgin
- Salsa, no sugar added
- Sesame oil, toasted
- Gluten-free soy sauce, such as tamari or Bragg Liquid Aminos
- Sriracha sauce (optional)
- Tomatoes, no salt added, whole or crushed, boxed
- Tomato sauce, no sugar added, boxed
- Vanilla bean, whole (optional)
- Vanilla extract, pure
- Vinegar, balsamic
- Vinegar, red wine
- Vinegar, sherry
- Wasabi paste (optional)
- Whey protein powder, grass-fed, vanilla

Pantry Items Stored in Refrigerator or Freezer

- Almond butter, unsalted raw or roasted
- Almond meal
- Almonds, whole, unsalted raw
- Cashews, unsalted raw
- Chia seeds, whole
- Coconut flakes, unsweetened
- Flaxseed, ground
- Hazelnuts, unsalted, roasted
- Horseradish, prepared
- Macadamia nuts, unsalted, lightly toasted
- Pine nuts
- Pistachios, unsalted roasted
- Pumpkin seeds, unsalted, raw or roasted
- Sesame seeds, toasted
- Walnuts, whole, unsalted raw
- Walnuts, chopped, unsalted toasted
- Walnut oil

Spices

- Ancho chili powder or cayenne pepper
- Bay leaves
- Black peppercorns
- Cinnamon, ground
- Cumin, ground
- Curry powder
- Fennel seeds
- Nutmeg, ground or whole
- Oregano, dried
- Paprika, sweet or smoked
- Red pepper flakes
- Rosemary, dried
- Sea salt
- Thyme, dried

Produce

- Apple, red (1)
- Avocados (5)
- Baby spinach (1 large bag)
- Basil, fresh (1 bunch)
- Bell pepper, green (1)
- Bell pepper, red (1)
- Bibb lettuce (2 heads) (optional)
- Carrots (1 medium bag)
- Celery (1 bunch)
- Chives, fresh (1 bunch)
- Chard, Swiss or rainbow (1 bunch)
- Cilantro, fresh (1 bunch)
- Collard greens (4 to 6 ounces)
- Cucumbers (2)
- Garlic (3 heads)
- Ginger (1 medium piece)
- Jalapeño or serrano peppers (4)
- Kale (1 large bunch)
- Lemons (6)
- Lettuce, Boston, red leaf, or romaine (2 heads)
- Limes (5)
- Onions, green (1 bunch)
- Onions, red (2)
- Onions, yellow (5)
- Oregano, fresh (1 bunch) (optional)
- Parsley, fresh flat-leaf (1 bunch)
- Rosemary, fresh (1 bunch) (optional)
- Squash, spaghetti (1 large and 1 small)
- Sweet potatoes (2 large)
- Thyme, fresh (1 bunch)
- Tomatillos (4)
- Tomatoes (5 to 6)
- Zucchini (1)

Protein

- Arctic char (or salmon) (four 6-ounce fillets)
- Bacon, applewood-smoked, nitrate-free (8-ounce package)
- Beef rib roast (one 3-rib slab, about 6 pounds)
- Chicken, whole fresh, quartered (one, 3½ pounds)
- Chicken breast, skinless, boneless (1 pound)
- Chicken, rotisserie, cooked (3 whole)
- Eggs (34)
- Eggs, hard-boiled (4)
- Ground beef or bison (1 pound)
- Ground pork or chicken (1 pound)
- Ground turkey (1 pound)
- Halibut steaks (four 6- to 8-ounce fillets)
- Pork shoulder roast, boneless (2½ pounds)
- Salmon, smoked, wild-caught (8 ounces)
- Steak, flat iron, flank, or top sirloin (1½ pounds)

Dairy Alternatives

- Almond milk, unsweetened
- Coconut milk, unsweetened

Refrigerated/Frozen Foods

- Blueberries, frozen (1 pound plus 3 cups)
- Strawberries, frozen (2 cups)

PLAN-AHEAD PREPARATIONS

When you're hungry, it's good to know that there's some prepared food waiting for you at home. Here are some suggestions for make-ahead foods that will also save you time making meals:

1. **Hard-Boiled Eggs:** If you're following a Paleo lifestyle, you can never have too many hard-boiled eggs on hand. Keep peeled, hard-boiled eggs in the refrigerator for a quick snack or an easy lunch like egg salad.
2. **Smoked Salmon Sushi Roll-Ups:** Make these in the morning or night before for a quick lunch.
3. **Nut butter:** Make your own nut butter (page 156) if unsalted, unprocessed versions are hard to find. This will come in handy for the Almond Butter Bites dessert.
4. **Desserts:** The Coconut Date "Blondies," Almond Butter Bites, Blueberry Macadamia Squares, and other desserts may be made ahead and stored in the refrigerator or freezer so you'll have something on hand when you need a sweet treat.
5. **Paleo Nut "Granola," Nutty Fruit Bars,** and **Chia Seed Pudding:** Make these recipes ahead to have on hand not only for breakfast but also for quick snacks.

CHAPTER FOUR

Week Two

WEEK TWO MEAL PLAN

Day One

Breakfast
Strawberry Shortcake Smoothie
Lunch
Salad made with leftover standing rib roast from dinner on Week One, Day 7, cherry tomatoes, and greens tossed with 1 tablespoon oil, 2 tablespoons horseradish sauce, and 2 teaspoons vinegar whisked together
Dinner
Tri-Colored Eggplant "Lasagna" with Sausage
Dessert
Almond Butter Cups

> **Daily Tip:** Some vegetables, like bell peppers, cucumbers, and carrots, are best when cut just before using.

Day Two

Breakfast
Maple-Fennel Breakfast Sausage with Scrambled Eggs
Lunch
Bunless Burgers with Sweet Potato Fries
Dinner
Stir-Fried Pork with Broccoli and Red Pepper
Dessert
Chocolate Chip Cookies

> **Daily Tip:** Never refrigerate tomatoes, as they will become mealy. Store them in a bowl at room temperature.

Day Three

Breakfast
Chorizo and Sweet Potato "Hash"
Lunch
Chicken, Kale, and Leek Soup using low-sodium broth or homemade Chicken Broth (page 158)
Dinner
Argentinean Skirt Steak with Chimichurri
Dessert
Chocolate-Cherry Bark

> **Daily Tip:** Listen to your body, not your mind, for what you crave. Then feed it appropriately with the wide range of healthful foods available to you. After a while, you'll find your body wanting vegetables and other healthful Paleo foods.

Day Four

Breakfast
Veggie Eggy Muffins with Caramelized Onions
Lunch
Steak Salad with Pumpkin Seeds and Creamy Cilantro-Lime Vinaigrette, using leftover skirt steak from dinner on Day 3
Dinner
Chard-Wrapped Arctic Char with Balsamic Glaze
Dessert
Coconut Vanilla Ice Cream

> **Daily Tip:** Eat a rainbow of nutrients. Load up on red, orange, yellow, green, blue, and purple vegetables to ensure you get your fill of antioxidants.

Day Five

Breakfast
Paleo Nut "Granola"
Lunch
Grilled Chicken "Caesar" Salad
Dinner
Asparagus Leek "Risotto" with Scallops
Dessert
Chocolate Coconut Truffles

> **Daily Tip:** Select produce carefully. Make sure the vegetables are brightly colored and perky, not brown or limp. If something doesn't look or smell fresh, skip it and shop elsewhere.

Day Six

Breakfast
Nutty Fruit Bars
Lunch
Roasted Butternut Squash and Pulled Chicken Soup
(or chicken from lunch on Day 5)
Dinner
Texas-Style Beef Chili
Dessert
Horchata Ice Pops

> **Daily Tip:** If you find nut butters made with raw nuts difficult to digest, soak and dry the nuts first. Soak almonds for eight hours, walnuts for four hours, and cashews for two hours. Allow the nuts to dry thoroughly before using, or use a dehydrator to speed up the process.

Day Seven

Breakfast
Chicken, Mushroom, Spinach, and Sage Omelet with Toasted Walnuts
Lunch
Leftover Veggie Eggy Muffins from breakfast on Day 4 with vegetables or a green salad
Dinner
Spicy Italian Fish Stew with Fennel
Dessert
Pumpkin Custard

Daily Tip: Headaches and fatigue may be symptoms of dehydration. Instead of reaching for an aspirin or other medication, drink a couple glasses of water.

WEEK TWO RECIPES

Breakfast

- Strawberry Shortcake Smoothie
- Maple-Fennel Breakfast Sausage with Scrambled Eggs
- Chorizo and Sweet Potato "Hash"
- Veggie Eggy Muffins with Caramelized Onions
- Paleo Nut "Granola"
- Nutty Fruit Bars
- Chicken, Mushroom, Spinach, and Sage Omelet with Toasted Walnuts

Lunch

- Bunless Burgers with Sweet Potato Fries
- Chicken, Kale, and Leek Soup
- Steak Salad with Pumpkin Seeds and Creamy Cilantro-Lime Vinaigrette
- Grilled Chicken "Caesar" Salad
- Roasted Butternut Squash and Pulled Chicken Soup

Dinner

- Tri-Colored Eggplant "Lasagna" with Sausage
- Stir-Fried Pork with Broccoli and Red Pepper
- Argentinean Skirt Steak with Chimichurri
- Chard-Wrapped Arctic Char with Balsamic Glaze
- Asparagus Leek "Risotto" with Scallops
- Texas-Style Beef Chili
- Spicy Italian Fish Stew with Fennel

Dessert

- Almond Butter Cups
- Chocolate Chip Cookies
- Chocolate-Cherry Bark
- Coconut Vanilla Ice Cream
- Chocolate Coconut Truffles
- Horchata Ice Pops
- Pumpkin Custard

WEEK TWO SHOPPING LIST

To prepare your meals for this week, purchase the following items in the quantities indicated:

Pantry Items

- Any missing pantry items and spices from Week One
- Almonds, unsalted, toasted (optional)
- Anchovies (optional)
- Chocolate, unsweetened
- Chocolate, unsweetened, dark
- Pumpkin puree (not pumpkin pie filling)

Produce

- Asparagus (1 small bunch)
- Avocados (3 to 4)
- Baby carrots (1 small bag)
- Baby spinach (1 bag)
- Basil, fresh (1 bunch)
- Bell peppers, green (2 to 3)
- Bell peppers, red (4 to 5)
- Bell peppers, yellow (2 to 3)

- Broccoli florets (1 bunch)
- Cauliflower (1 head)
- Chard, Swiss or rainbow (1 bunch)
- Cilantro, fresh (1 bunch)
- Cucumber (1)
- Eggplants (2 large)
- Fennel (1 bulb with fronds)
- Garlic (2 heads)
- Greens, mixed (1 bag)
- Jalapeño or serrano peppers (2 to 3)
- Kale (1 bunch)
- Leeks (2)
- Lemon (1)
- Lettuce, Bibb (1 head)
- Lettuce, romaine (1 head)
- Lime (1)
- Mushrooms, cremini or button (2 cups)
- Onion, red (1)
- Onions, green (2)
- Onions, yellow (4)
- Parsley, fresh, flat-leaf (1 bunch)
- Sage, fresh (8 leaves)
- Squash, butternut (1 medium to large)
- Sweet potatoes (4)
- Thyme, fresh (1 bunch) (optional)
- Tomatoes (2)
- Tomatoes, cherry (1 pint)
- Zucchini (2)

Protein

- Arctic char (four 6-ounce fillets)
- Chicken breast, boneless, skinless (four 4- to 6-ounce pieces)
- Chorizo (1 pound)
- Eggs (30)
- Ground beef chuck or bison (2 pounds)
- Ground pork or chicken (2 pounds)
- Italian sausage (1 pound)
- Pork tenderloin (1 pound)
- Scallops (1½ pound)
- Steak, skirt or flat iron (2½ to 3 pounds)
- Tilapia or other whitefish fillets (1 pound)

Dairy Alternatives

- Almond milk, unsweetened
- Coconut milk, unsweetened

Refrigerated/Frozen Foods

- Strawberries, frozen (2½ cups)

PLAN-AHEAD PREPARATIONS

When you're hungry, it's good to know that there's some prepared food waiting for you at home. Here are some suggestions for make-ahead foods that will also save you time making meals:

1. **Hard-boiled eggs:** If you're following a Paleo lifestyle, you can never have too many hard-boiled eggs on hand. Keep peeled, hard-boiled eggs in the refrigerator for a quick snack or an easy lunch like egg salad.
2. **Smoked Salmon Sushi Roll-Ups:** Make these in the morning or night before for a quick lunch.
3. **Guacamole:** When making guacamole ahead of time, place a piece of plastic wrap directly on the surface of the guacamole to keep it from turning brown. Cover it well and store it in the refrigerator.
4. **Nut butter:** Make your own nut butter (page 156) if unsalted, unprocessed versions are hard to find. This will come in handy for the Almond Butter Bites dessert.
5. **Desserts:** The Chocolate Chip Cookies, Chocolate-Cherry Bark, and Coconut Vanilla Ice Cream desserts may be made ahead and stored in the refrigerator or freezer so you'll have something on hand when you need a sweet treat.
6. **Paleo Nut "Granola," Nutty Fruit Bars,** and **Pumpkin Custard:** Make these recipes ahead to have on hand not only for breakfast but also for quick snacks.

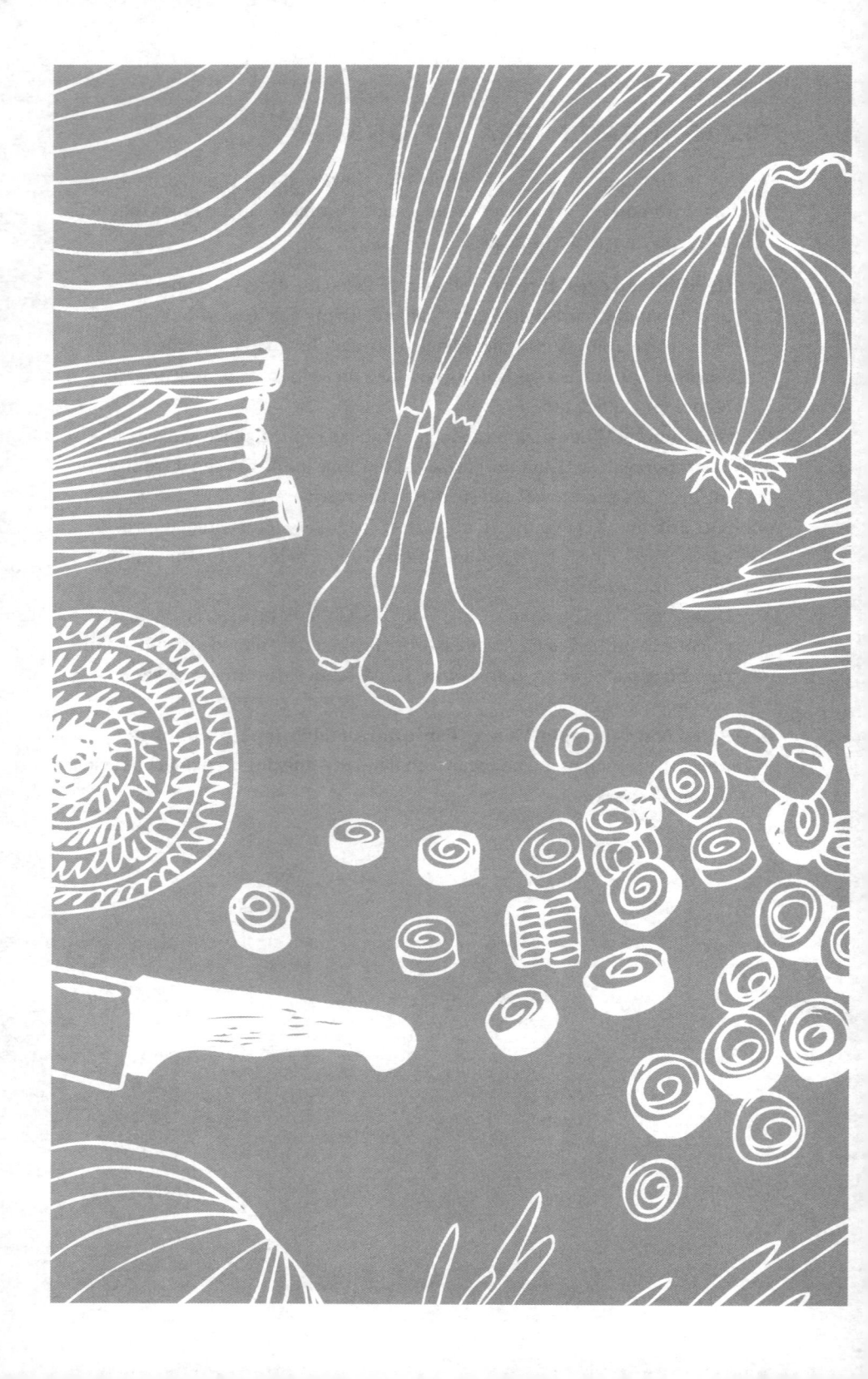

CHAPTER FIVE

Week Three

WEEK THREE MEAL PLAN

Day One

Breakfast
Spanish Sweet Potato Tortilla
Lunch
Beef "Tacos" with Salsa and Guacamole
Dinner
Maple-Glazed Pork Chops with Roasted Brussels Sprouts, Bacon, and Walnuts
Dessert: Quick and Easy Microwave Brownie

Day Two

Breakfast
Poached Eggs "Florentine"
Lunch
Leftover Texas-Style Beef Chili from dinner on Week Two, Day 6, and a small green salad or sliced cucumber with guacamole
Dinner
Spanish Chicken with Romesco Sauce
Dessert
Paleo "Cheesecake"

> **Daily Tip:** Ditch the plastic bags from the grocery stores and use reusable mesh or other special produce bags to let produce breathe and maintain freshness.

Day Three

Breakfast
Paleo Nut "Granola" with 1 or 2 hard-boiled eggs
Lunch
Tuna Salad–Stuffed Tomatoes
Dinner
Lamb Kebabs with Parsley-Mint Sauce
Dessert
Chocolate-Cherry Bark

> **Daily Tip:** Prevent nuts from going rancid by storing them in the refrigerator or freezer in airtight plastic bags. Nut oils also last longer when stored in the refrigerator.

Day Four

Breakfast
Blueberry Power Breakfast Smoothie
Lunch
Fried Cauliflower "Rice" with Shrimp
Dinner
Lemon-Poached Salmon with Roasted Balsamic-Glazed Kale and Cherry Tomatoes
Dessert
Very Berry Granita

> **Daily Tip:** Massages can be great for sore muscles. Always stretch after exercising and soak in an Epsom salt bath for additional detoxing and muscle relaxation.

Day Five

Breakfast
Nutty Fruit Bar with 1 or 2 hard-boiled eggs
Lunch
Salmon Burgers with Carrot-Cabbage Slaw
Dinner
Tri-Colored Eggplant "Lasagna" with Sausage and a small green salad
Dessert
Chocolate Coconut Truffles

> **Daily Tip:** If your schedule permits, try to exercise first thing in the morning. Even just fifteen minutes of activity will invigorate you, and the residual effects will boost your metabolism for the rest of the day.

Day Six

Breakfast
Veggie Eggy Muffins with Caramelized Onions (leftover or made fresh)
Lunch
Gazpacho with Crab
Dinner
Mustard-Crusted Chicken Thighs and Garlicky Greens
Dessert
Chia Seed Pudding

> **Daily Tip:** Suffering from foot or joint pain? It could be your sneakers! It sounds strange, but consider scaling *down* your shoe cushioning. Though it takes some getting used to, minimal and barefoot-style shoes can help strengthen ankle, calf, and hip muscles to improve leg strength and posture to prevent joint damage. Minimal shoes also make sporadic and plyometric movements like jumping, sprinting, and lunging easier.

Day Seven

Breakfast
Blueberry-Almond Paleo Pancakes

Lunch
Vegetable salad using leftover chicken thighs from dinner on Day 6 with oil and vinegar

Dinner
Classic Beef Stew with Sweet Potatoes

Dessert
Coconut Vanilla Ice Cream

> **Daily Tip:** Coconut, avocado, grape-seed, and some olive oils have a higher smoking point than less refined olive and nut oils, and are therefore best used in cooking, searing, roasting, and baking. Reserve specialty walnut, avocado, hazelnut, and flaxseed oils as finishing oils to add flavor more nutrition to your salads and raw dishes; cooking and high heat can strip the healthy properties from these oils.

WEEK THREE RECIPES

Breakfast

- Spanish Sweet Potato Tortilla
- Poached Eggs "Florentine"
- Paleo Nut "Granola"
- Blueberry Power Breakfast Smoothie
- Nutty Fruit Bar
- Veggie Eggy Muffins with Caramelized Onions
- Blueberry-Almond Paleo Pancakes

Lunch

- Beef "Tacos" with Salsa and Guacamole
- Tuna Salad–Stuffed Tomatoes
- Fried Cauliflower "Rice" with Shrimp
- Salmon Burgers with Carrot-Cabbage Slaw
- Gazpacho with Crab

Dinner

- Maple-Glazed Pork Chops with Roasted Brussels Sprouts, Bacon, and Walnuts
- Spanish Chicken with Romesco Sauce
- Lamb Kebabs with Parsley-Mint Sauce
- Lemon-Poached Salmon with Roasted Balsamic-Glazed Kale and Cherry Tomatoes
- Tri-Colored Eggplant "Lasagna" with Sausage
- Mustard-Crusted Chicken Thighs and Garlicky Greens
- Classic Beef Stew with Sweet Potatoes

Dessert

- Quick and Easy Microwave Brownie
- Paleo "Cheesecake"
- Chocolate-Cherry Bark
- Very Berry Granita
- Chocolate Coconut Truffles
- Chia Seed Pudding
- Coconut Vanilla Ice Cream

WEEK THREE SHOPPING LIST

To prepare your meals for this week, purchase the following items in the quantities indicated:

Pantry Items

- Any missing pantry items and spices from Week One
- Red peppers, roasted

Produce

- Arugula (1 bunch) (optional)
- Avocados (2 to 3)
- Baby spinach (1 bag)
- Basil, fresh (1 bunch)
- Bell peppers, red (2 to 3)
- Bell peppers, yellow (2 to 3)
- Berries, mixed (4 cups)
- Brussels sprouts (1 to 1½ pounds)
- Cabbage, red (1 head or 2 cups shredded)
- Carrots (1 large bag)

- Cauliflower (1 head)
- Chives, fresh (1 bunch) (optional)
- Cilantro, fresh (2 bunches)
- Collard greens (1 large bunch)
- Cucumber (1)
- Eggplants (2 large)
- Garlic (2 heads)
- Jalapeño pepper (1)
- Kale (1 bunch)
- Lemons (5)
- Lettuce, Bibb or romaine (1 head)
- Limes (3)
- Mint, fresh (1 bunch)
- Mushrooms, cremini or button (1 cup)
- Mustard greens or Swiss chard (1 bunch)
- Onions, green (1 bunch)
- Onions, red (3)
- Onions, yellow (3)
- Parsley, fresh, flat-leaf (1 bunch)
- Snow peas (1 cup)
- Sweet potatoes (6)
- Thyme, fresh (1 bunch)
- Tomatoes (6)
- Tomatoes, cherry (1 pint)
- Tomatoes, plum (8)
- Zucchini (1)

Protein

- Bacon, nitrate-free, thick cut (1 package)
- Beef stew meat (1¼ pounds)
- Chicken breasts, bone-in (4)
- Chicken thighs, bone-in (4 large or 8 small)
- Chicken, rotisserie, cooked, if needed
- Crabmeat, lump (2 cups)
- Eggs (27)
- Eggs, hard-boiled (6)
- Ground beef chuck or bison (1 pound)
- Italian sausage (1 pound)
- Leg of lamb, boneless (1 pound)
- Pork chops (4 large)
- Salmon, wild-caught, fresh (four 4- to 6-ounce fillets)
- Salmon, wild-caught, canned (14.5 ounces)
- Shrimp (2 cups)
- Tuna, canned in water (one, 5 to 6 ounces)

Dairy Alternatives

- Almond milk, unsweetened
- Coconut milk, unsweetened

Refrigerated/Frozen Foods

- Blueberries, frozen (3 cups)

PLAN-AHEAD PREPARATIONS

When you're hungry, it's good to know that there's some prepared food waiting for you at home. Here are some suggestions for make-ahead foods that will also save you time making meals:

1. **Hard-boiled eggs:** If you're following a Paleo lifestyle, you can never have too many hard-boiled eggs on hand. Keep peeled, hard-boiled eggs in the refrigerator for a quick snack or an easy lunch like egg salad.
2. **Smoked Salmon Sushi Roll-Ups:** Make these in the morning or night before for a quick lunch.
3. **Guacamole:** When making guacamole ahead of time, place a piece of plastic wrap directly on the surface of the guacamole to keep it from turning brown. Cover it well and store it in the refrigerator.
4. **Nut butter:** Make your own nut butter (page 156) if unsalted, unprocessed versions are hard to find. This will come in handy for the Almond Butter Bites dessert.
5. **Desserts:** The Chocolate-Cherry Bark, Paleo "Cheesecake," Chocolate Coconut Truffles, and other desserts may be made ahead and stored in the refrigerator or freezer so you'll have something on hand when you need a sweet treat.
6. **Paleo Nut "Granola," Nutty Fruit Bars,** and **Chia Seed Pudding:** Make these recipes ahead to have on hand not only for breakfast but also for quick snacks.
7. **Romesco Sauce:** This quick and easy sauce can be made ahead to pair with the Spanish Chicken recipe on Day 2.

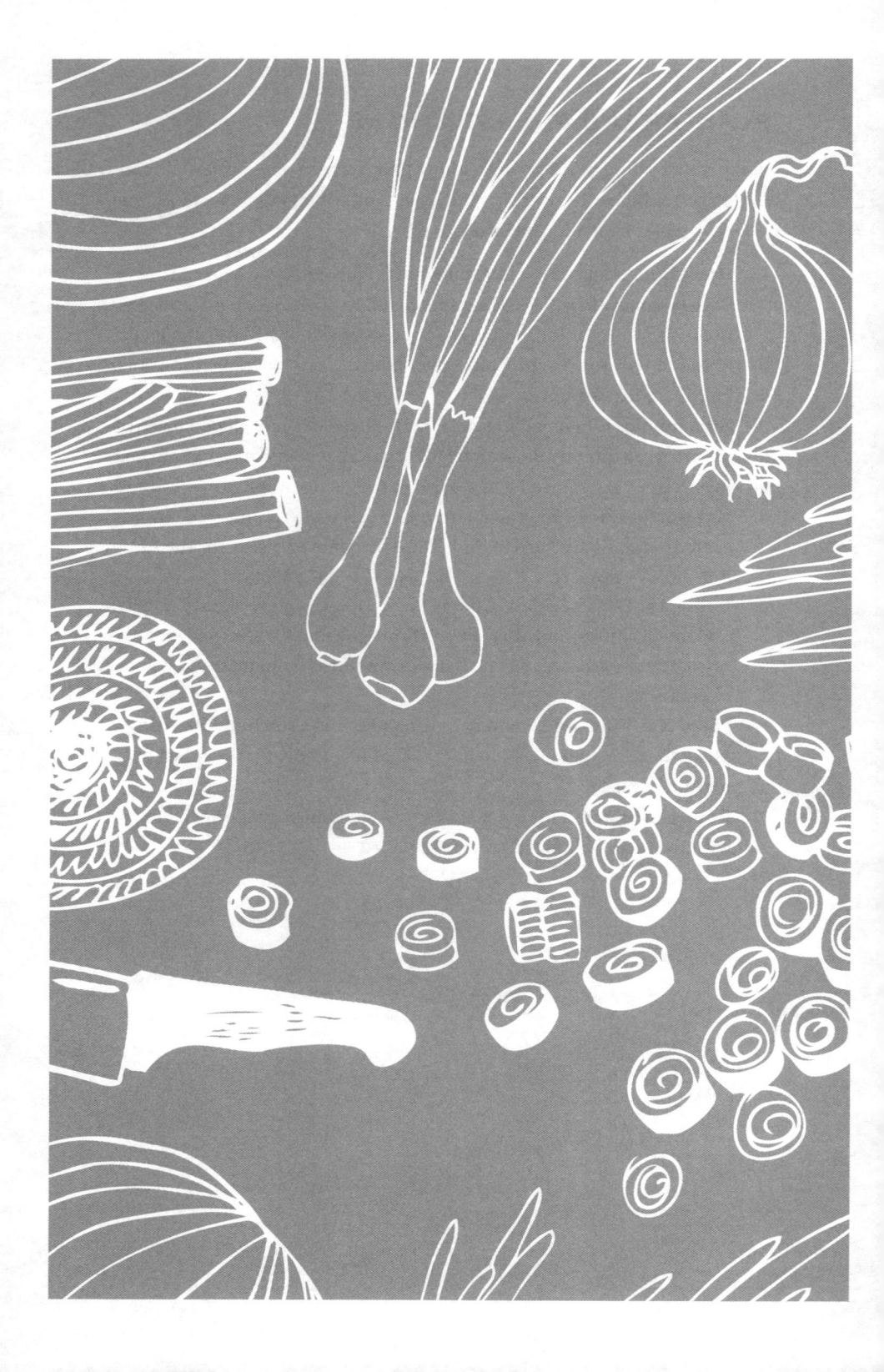

PART THREE

Paleo Diet Recipes

CHAPTER SIX BREAKFAST

CHAPTER SEVEN LUNCH

CHAPTER EIGHT DINNER

CHAPTER NINE DESSERT

CHAPTER TEN PANTRY RECIPES

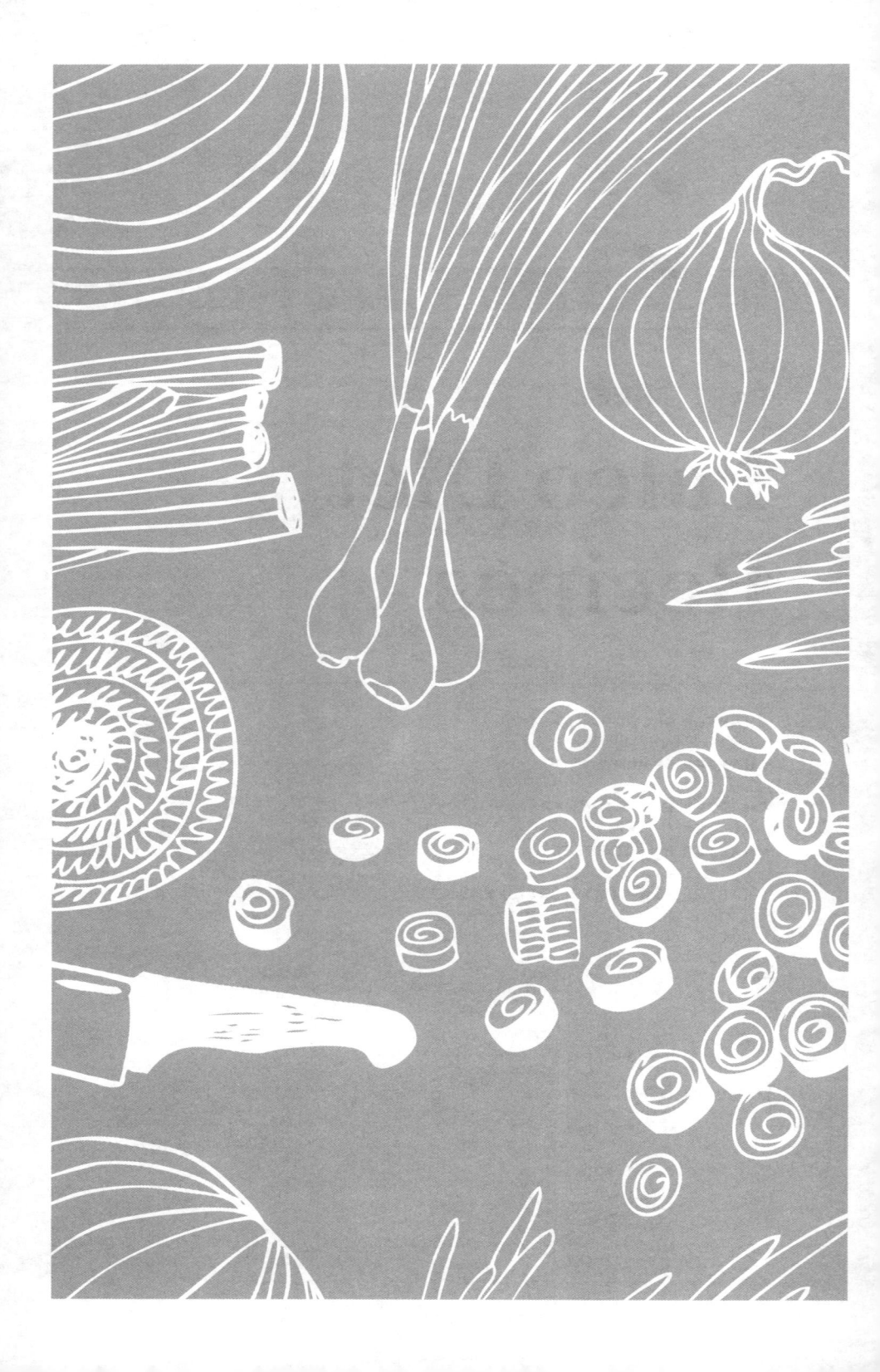

CHAPTER SIX

Breakfast

STRAWBERRY SHORTCAKE SMOOTHIE

BLUEBERRY POWER BREAKFAST SMOOTHIE

"NUTELLA" SMOOTHIE

PALEO NUT "GRANOLA"

NUTTY FRUIT BARS

VEGGIE EGGY MUFFINS WITH CARAMELIZED ONIONS

BLUEBERRY-ALMOND PALEO PANCAKES

FRITTATA WITH BACON, COLLARD GREENS, AND SCALLIONS

CHICKEN, MUSHROOM, SPINACH, AND SAGE OMELET WITH TOASTED WALNUTS

LOX, EGGS, AND ONION SCRAMBLE

MAPLE-FENNEL BREAKFAST SAUSAGE WITH SCRAMBLED EGGS

CHORIZO AND SWEET POTATO "HASH"

SPANISH SWEET POTATO TORTILLA

POACHED EGGS "FLORENTINE"

POACHED EGGS WITH SPICY TOMATO SAUCE

Strawberry Shortcake Smoothie

SERVES 2

Like dessert for breakfast, this antioxidant, omega-3-rich smoothie will power up your day. Swap almonds for the cashews, if desired.

2½ CUPS FROZEN STRAWBERRIES
2 CUPS UNSWEETENED ALMOND MILK, CHILLED
¼ CUP RAW OR ROASTED UNSALTED CASHEWS
2 SERVINGS VANILLA-FLAVORED GRASS-FED WHEY PROTEIN POWDER
2 TABLESPOONS GROUND FLAXSEEDS

1. Place all the ingredients in a blender and process for 30 seconds on high speed.

2. Pour the smoothie into two glasses and serve immediately.

Blueberry Power Breakfast Smoothie

SERVES 2

Smoothies are a quick and easy way to power up your day. Adding a handful of mild baby spinach boosts the antioxidant factor without adding any noticeable changes to the flavor. Maca, a root vegetable grown in Peru, has energy-boosting properties and is great when you're trying to avoid or limit caffeine, but just a touch goes a long way. When selecting protein powder, look for brands without added sugar or preservatives, and powders that are made from grass-fed and pastured cows, if possible, for extra omega-3 fatty acids.

2½ CUPS FROZEN BLUEBERRIES
1 CUP BABY SPINACH LEAVES
2 CUPS UNSWEETENED COCONUT WATER, CHILLED
2 SERVINGS VANILLA-FLAVORED GRASS-FED WHEY PROTEIN POWDER (OR HEMP PROTEIN POWDER)
1 TABLESPOON UNSALTED RAW OR ROASTED ALMOND BUTTER
1 TEASPOON MACA POWDER (OPTIONAL)

1. Put all of the ingredients in a blender. Blend for 30 seconds on high speed.

2. Pour the smoothie into two glasses and serve immediately.

"Nutella" Smoothie

SERVES 2

Nothing beats chocolate with hazelnut. With naturally sweet dates and anti-inflammatory cacao, you can skip the sugary spread for this Paleo-friendly version.

5 PITTED MEDJOOL DATES
¼ CUP UNSALTED ROASTED HAZELNUTS
1 TABLESPOON RAW CACAO POWDER OR UNSWEETENED COCOA
2 CUPS UNSWEETENED ALMOND MILK, CHILLED
2 SCOOPS VANILLA-FLAVORED GRASS-FED WHEY PROTEIN POWDER
½ CUP ICE
1 TABLESPOON GROUND FLAXSEEDS (OPTIONAL)

1. Place all the ingredients in a blender and process for 30 seconds on high speed.

2. Pour the smoothie into two glasses and serve immediately.

Paleo Nut "Granola"

MAKES 4 TO 5 CUPS

Missing cereal? Try this nut granola for a healthier, more satisfying treat that will stave off hunger all morning long. Serve it with almond or coconut milk, berries, and hard-boiled eggs on the side for extra protein, if desired. Store leftover granola in an airtight container in the refrigerator for about a month. This recipe also pairs great with Chia Seed Pudding (page 138).

1 CUP SLICED RAW UNSALTED ALMONDS
1 CUP CHOPPED RAW UNSALTED WALNUTS
½ CUP RAW UNSALTED PUMPKIN SEEDS
3 TABLESPOONS GROUND FLAXSEED
½ CUP UNSWEETENED COCONUT FLAKES
½ CUP COCONUT OIL, MELTED
½ CUP RAW HONEY OR GRADE B PURE MAPLE SYRUP
1½ TEASPOONS GROUND CINNAMON
¼ TEASPOON SEA SALT
1 CUP DRIED UNSWEETENED CRANBERRIES, CHERRIES, AND/OR BLUEBERRIES

1. Preheat the oven to 300°F.

2. Combine all the ingredients except the dried fruit in a large microwave-safe bowl and mix well. Microwave the granola for 20 seconds if honey makes the mixture too thick to mix.

3. Spread the mixture onto a baking sheet lined with foil or lightly greased with coconut oil.

4. Bake the granola for 20 to 25 minutes, stirring occasionally to prevent burning.

5. Remove the granola from the oven and stir in the dried fruit.

Nutty Fruit Bars

MAKES 20 BARS

These granola-like bars are great for an on-the-go breakfast, quick snack, or even dessert.

1¼ CUPS WHOLE RAW UNSALTED ALMONDS
¼ CUP ROASTED UNSALTED PISTACHIOS
½ CUP WHOLE UNSALTED WALNUTS
¾ CUP ALMOND MEAL
½ CUP UNSWEETENED COCONUT FLAKES
½ CUP DRIED UNSWEETENED CHERRIES, FINELY CHOPPED
½ CUP RAW HONEY
¼ CUP WALNUT OIL
1 EGG WHITE
1 TABLESPOON GROUND FLAXSEED
2 TEASPOONS PURE VANILLA EXTRACT
½ TEASPOON GROUND CINNAMON

1. Preheat the oven to 325°F.

2. Combine the almonds, pistachios, and walnuts in a food processor. Cover and pulse until they are finely chopped; then transfer the nuts to a large mixing bowl.

3. Add the remaining ingredients to the nuts and mix well.

4. Spread the mixture very firmly in an even layer in a foil-lined 9-by-9-inch baking pan, allowing some of the foil to line the sides.

5. Bake the mixture for 20 minutes or until it is a deep golden brown.

6. Use the foil edges to transfer the baked square to a wire rack. Allow it to cool completely.

7. Transfer the square to a cutting board. Use a long sharp knife to cut the square into 20 bars. Store the bars in the refrigerator for up to 2 weeks.

Veggie Eggy Muffins with Caramelized Onions

SERVES 8

These egg "muffins" are great for quick breakfasts or even a light lunch when paired with a side salad. Store leftover chopped zucchini and peppers in the refrigerator for salad add-ins or in the freezer for soups and chili.

3 TABLESPOONS EXTRA-VIRGIN OLIVE OIL
1 YELLOW ONION, SLICED
1 CUP FINELY CHOPPED CREMINI OR BUTTON MUSHROOMS
½ CUP FINELY DICED RED BELL PEPPER
½ CUP FINELY DICED ZUCCHINI
¼ TEASPOON SEA SALT
¼ TEASPOON FRESHLY GROUND BLACK PEPPER
8 EGGS, BEATEN
½ TEASPOON DRIED OREGANO
½ AVOCADO, PEELED, SEEDED, AND DICED (OPTIONAL)
¼ CUP SALSA OR HOT SAUCE (OPTIONAL)

1. Preheat the oven to 350°F.

2. Grease an 8-cup muffin pan or line it with paper liners.

3. Heat 2 tablespoons of the olive oil in a large skillet over medium heat. Add the onion and cook it until it is tender and caramelized, stirring often, about 10 minutes. Remove the onion from the pan and divide it evenly among muffin cups.

4. Add the remaining 1 tablespoon of olive oil, mushrooms, bell pepper, and zucchini, and cook for 5 to 7 minutes, or until the vegetables are tender and the mushrooms release their liquid. Season the mixture with salt and pepper.

5. Turn off the heat. Add the eggs and oregano, stirring gently. Divide the vegetable-egg mixture between the muffin cups.

continued ▶

Veggie Eggy Muffins with Caramelized Onions *continued* ▶

6. Bake the muffins until the eggs are set in the middle and browned on top, 15 to 20 minutes.

7. Remove the muffins from oven and allow them to cool for 5 minutes.

8. Serve the muffins warm with chopped avocado and salsa or hot sauce (if using). Wrap leftover muffins in plastic wrap and store them in the refrigerator for up to 5 days or in the freezer for 2 to 3 months.

Blueberry-Almond Paleo Pancakes

SERVES 4

Just because you're following the Paleo lifestyle doesn't mean you can't have pancakes. This gluten-free version is packed with blueberries for extra nutrients. Serve pancakes with eggs and/or bacon or sausage for a more balanced, protein-rich breakfast.

1½ CUPS ALMOND MEAL
½ TEASPOON BAKING SODA
½ TEASPOON BAKING POWDER
PINCH OF SEA SALT
4 EGGS
¼ CUP UNSWEETENED ALMOND MILK
¼ CUP COCONUT OIL, MELTED, PLUS 1 TABLESPOON FOR COOKING
1 TEASPOON PURE VANILLA EXTRACT
¼ CUP FRESH OR FROZEN BLUEBERRIES
4 TABLESPOONS GRADE B PURE MAPLE SYRUP, WARMED (OPTIONAL)

1. In a medium bowl, combine the almond meal, baking soda, baking powder, and salt.

2. In a separate bowl, whisk together the eggs, almond milk, ¼ cup of the coconut oil, and vanilla.

3. Whisk the dry ingredients into the wet ingredients. Fold in the blueberries.

4. Heat the remaining 1 tablespoon of coconut oil in a large skillet or griddle over medium-high heat. Use 3 tablespoons of pancake batter to make each pancake on the skillet or griddle. Do not overcrowd the pan.

5. Cook the pancakes until they are set and browned on the bottom, about 3 minutes. Flip the pancakes and cook through, another 2 minutes.

6. Serve the pancakes with 1 tablespoon of grade B pure maple syrup (if using).

Frittata with Bacon, Collard Greens, and Scallions

SERVES 6

Rich and satisfying, this nutrient-rich frittata is a great way to start your day. Portion out and refrigerate leftover frittata slices for a quick breakfast or light lunch paired with a small green salad.

8 OUNCES NITRATE-FREE APPLEWOOD-SMOKED BACON, CUT INTO ½-INCH PIECES
¾ CUP THINLY SLICED SCALLIONS
3 TO 4 CUPS (4 TO 6 OUNCES) STEMMED AND COARSELY CHOPPED COLLARD GREENS
12 EGGS
½ TEASPOON SEA SALT
¼ TEASPOON FRESHLY GROUND BLACK PEPPER
½ CUP COLD WATER
THINLY SLICED CHIVES, SALSA OR HOT SAUCE, AND SLICED AVOCADO, FOR GARNISH (OPTIONAL)

1. Preheat the oven to 350°F.

2. In a 12-inch ovenproof skillet over medium-high heat, cook the bacon until crisp, about 5 minutes. Using a slotted spoon, transfer the bacon to paper towels to drain. Pour the bacon drippings into a bowl and reserve.

3. Return 2 tablespoons of drippings to the skillet. Add the scallions and sauté them over medium heat until tender, about 3 minutes.

4. Add two-thirds of the greens and toss until they are wilted and tender, about 2 minutes. Transfer the greens to a plate and allow them to cool slightly.

5. Beat the eggs, salt, pepper, and water in a large bowl until blended. Whisk in the remaining greens and the bacon.

6. Heat 1 tablespoon of the reserved drippings in the skillet over medium heat. Store any remaining bacon drippings in the refrigerator for future use.

7. Pour the egg mixture into the skillet and top it evenly with the reserved cooked greens. Cook the egg mixture over medium heat until the frittata is just set at edges, about 10 minutes.

8. Transfer the frittata to the oven and bake it until it is set and golden, 17 to 20 minutes.

9. Slide a spatula under and around frittata to loosen it, and then slide it onto a platter. Let it cool for 30 minutes.

10. Slice the frittata into 6 wedges. Serve immediately with garnishes (if using).

Chicken, Mushroom, Spinach, and Sage Omelet with Toasted Walnuts

SERVES 2

This savory and satisfying omelet will put your leftover chicken to great use. Mushrooms pack extra vitamin D, while the walnuts boost your omega-3 intake.

3 TABLESPOONS COCONUT OIL
¼ CUP CHOPPED WALNUTS
3 TABLESPOONS DICED RED ONION
1 CUP SLICED CREMINI OR BUTTON MUSHROOMS
½ TEASPOON SEA SALT
¼ TEASPOON FRESHLY GROUND BLACK PEPPER
4 OUNCES LEFTOVER ROTISSERIE OR COOKED CHICKEN, SHREDDED
8 SAGE LEAVES, THINLY SLICED
1 CUP BABY SPINACH
4 EGGS, BEATEN
3 TABLESPOONS CHOPPED FRESH FLAT-LEAF PARSLEY OR FRESH THYME LEAVES (OPTIONAL)

1. In a large skillet, cook 2 tablespoons of coconut oil and the walnuts over medium heat until the oil is fragrant and the walnuts are golden toasted, 2 to 3 minutes.

2. Add the onion and mushrooms, and cook until the onion is tender and the mushrooms release their juices and begin to brown, 5 to 6 minutes.

3. Season the mixture with salt and pepper; then add the chicken, sage, and spinach and cook until warmed and the spinach has wilted, about 2 minutes. Remove the entire vegetable mixture from the pan and set it aside.

4. Add the remaining 1 tablespoon of oil and pour in the eggs. Cook the eggs for 1 minute until the bottom begins to set. Tilt the skillet, lifting the edges of the omelet with a spatula to let the uncooked egg flow underneath. Cook until the eggs begin to set.

5. Spoon the vegetable mixture over half of the omelet. Using the spatula, fold the other half over the filling and allow the egg to cook for 1 minute.

6. Cut the omelet in half and divide it between two plates. Serve the omelet with the parsley or thyme (if using).

Lox, Eggs, and Onion Scramble

SERVES 2

Also known as smoked salmon, lox is a classic breakfast staple and a great way to add more heart-healthful fish to your diet. Some smoked salmon versions are saltier than others, so choose carefully.

2 TABLESPOONS EXTRA-VIRGIN OLIVE OIL
1 YELLOW ONION, DICED
4 OUNCES SLICED WILD-CAUGHT SMOKED SALMON, CUT INTO LARGE STRIPS
4 EGGS, BEATEN
¼ TEASPOON FRESHLY GROUND BLACK PEPPER
3 TABLESPOONS CHOPPED FRESH CHIVES

1. Heat the olive oil over medium heat in a large skillet. Add the onion and cook until lightly browned, about 3 minutes.

2. Reduce heat to low. Add the salmon and eggs, and cook until the eggs are set but creamy, stirring frequently, about 3 to 4 minutes.

3. Season the salmon and eggs with pepper and top with the chives. Serve hot.

Maple-Fennel Breakfast Sausage with Scrambled Eggs

SERVES 4

Craving a classic diner breakfast? Making your own sausage controls the ingredients and sodium for a "cleaner" version. The grated zucchini addition is a great way to sneak in some extra vegetables.

½ TEASPOON SEA SALT
½ TEASPOON FRESHLY GROUND BLACK PEPPER
1 TEASPOON FENNEL SEEDS
1 POUND GROUND PORK OR CHICKEN
1 CUP GRATED ZUCCHINI
2 TABLESPOONS GRADE B PURE MAPLE SYRUP
2 TABLESPOONS EXTRA-VIRGIN OLIVE OIL
8 EGGS, BEATEN

1. In a large bowl, combine the salt, pepper, and fennel. Add the pork and zucchini and mix well to combine.

2. Add the maple syrup and gently mix the meat again.

3. Shape the meat into 4 patties, each 2 to 3 inches wide and ½ inch thick.

4. In a large skillet, heat the olive oil over medium-high heat. Cook the patties until they are browned, 4 to 5 minutes per side. Transfer sausage patties to a paper towel–lined plate.

5. In the same skillet, add the eggs and cook over low heat until they are set but creamy, stirring frequently, about 3 to 4 minutes.

6. Serve the eggs with the sausage patties.

Chorizo and Sweet Potato "Hash"

SERVES 4

This hearty and multicolored skillet breakfast will power up your day. Save leftovers in the refrigerator (up to three days) or in the freezer (for up to two months) for a quick breakfast, lunch, or even light dinner.

2 SWEET POTATOES, DICED (ABOUT 4 CUPS)
2 TABLESPOONS COCONUT OR EXTRA-VIRGIN OLIVE OIL
1 POUND CHORIZO, REMOVED FROM CASING
1 CUP DICED YELLOW ONION
1 RED BELL PEPPER, DICED
1 GREEN BELL PEPPER, DICED
1 GARLIC CLOVE, MINCED
½ TEASPOON MINCED SEEDED JALAPEÑO PEPPER (OPTIONAL)
1 TEASPOON GROUND CUMIN
1 AVOCADO, PEELED, SEEDED, AND SLICED
½ CUP CHOPPED CILANTRO (OPTIONAL)

1. Pierce the sweet potatoes with a knife and place them in a microwave-safe bowl with a splash of water. Microwave the sweet potatoes on high heat until they are tender, about 6 minutes.

2. Allow the sweet potatoes to cool; then slice them into ¼-inch-thick pieces and set them aside.

3. Heat 1 tablespoon of the oil in a large skillet and add the chorizo. Cook, breaking up chunks with a wooden spoon, until all the meat is browned, 8 to 10 minutes. Transfer the chorizo to a paper towel–lined plate.

4. Add the remaining 1 tablespoon of oil and the onions to the skillet. Cook until the onion is soft and translucent, stirring to collect chorizo drippings, about 2 minutes.

5. Add the bell peppers, garlic, and jalapeño (if using). Cook until the vegetables are tender, 5 to 6 minutes, stirring occasionally.

6. Add the chorizo, sweet potato, and cumin, and cook until heated through, stirring to combine.

7. Serve the hash immediately with the avocado slices and cilantro (if using).

Spanish Sweet Potato Tortilla

SERVES 8

This Spanish-style omelet (aka tortilla) swaps out white potatoes for beta-carotene-rich sweet potatoes. Save extra slices in the refrigerator for up to 3 days for quick breakfasts, snacks, and light lunches throughout the week. Avocado slices add an extra dose of healthy fat.

4 OR 5 MEDIUM SWEET POTATOES (ABOUT 1¾ POUND), PEELED AND HALVED LENGTHWISE
½ TEASPOON SEA SALT
½ TEASPOON FRESHLY GROUND BLACK PEPPER
¼ CUP EXTRA-VIRGIN OLIVE OIL
1 RED ONION, FINELY DICED
6 EGGS
AVOCADO SLICES (OPTIONAL)
CHOPPED CHIVES (OPTIONAL)

1. Using a very sharp knife or mandoline, slice the sweet potatoes as thinly as possible. Season them with ¼ teaspoon of both salt and pepper.

2. Heat the olive oil in a large, heavy skillet at least 1½ inches deep over medium-high heat. When the oil is hot, evenly distribute the sweet potatoes in the skillet.

3. Fry the sweet potatoes until they are tender and browned, about 10 minutes, flipping occasionally. Transfer the sweet potatoes to paper towel–lined plate.

4. Drain the oil, if necessary, leaving 2 tablespoons in the skillet. Add the onion and cook over medium heat until soft and translucent, about 2 minutes.

5. In a large bowl, beat the eggs with the remaining ¼ teaspoon of salt and pepper. Carefully fold in the sweet potatoes and pour the mixture into skillet with the onion.

6. Cook the egg mixture until it is set on the bottom and the tortilla moves around when the skillet is shaken, 8 to 10 minutes.

7. Invert the tortilla onto a large flat plate and slide it back into the skillet, bottom-side up. Cook until the tortilla is set, about 3 minutes.

8. To serve, cut the tortilla into 8 wedges and serve it with sliced avocado and chopped fresh chives (if using).

Poached Eggs "Florentine"

SERVES 2

This Paleo-friendly dish has been modeled after classic eggs Florentine, which normally consists of poached eggs and buttery hollandaise sauce atop spinach and English muffins. Here, fresh lemon juice, bacon, and tomato slices stand in for the bread and sauce for a fresh and starch-free, yet still hearty, option.

4 STRIPS NITRATE-FREE BACON
5 CUPS BABY SPINACH
¼ TEASPOON SEA SALT
¼ TEASPOON FRESHLY GROUND BLACK PEPPER, PLUS MORE
   FOR GARNISH
⅛ TEASPOON GROUND NUTMEG
1 TABLESPOON FRESH LEMON JUICE
1 TEASPOON APPLE CIDER VINEGAR
2 EGGS
2 BEEFSTEAK OR VINE-RIPENED TOMATOES, CUT INTO
   1-INCH-THICK SLICES

1. In a large skillet over medium-high heat, cook the bacon strips until they are slightly crisp, 5 to 7 minutes, flipping once. Using tongs, transfer the bacon to a paper towel–lined plate. Drain off the bacon grease into a small bowl, leaving 1 to 2 tablespoons in the skillet. Refrigerate the extra grease for later use.

2. Reduce the heat to medium and add the spinach, cooking until just wilted, about 30 seconds to 1 minute. Use tongs to coat the spinach in bacon grease.

3. Toss the spinach with salt, pepper, nutmeg, and lemon juice; then set it aside.

4. Fill a medium saucepan with 3 inches of water and bring to a boil. Reduce the heat to a simmer and add the vinegar.

5. One at a time, crack each egg into a small bowl and slide it into the pot. Cook the eggs until they are just runny, about 3 minutes. Remove the eggs with a slotted spoon.

6. To serve, divide the tomato slices between two plates. Top the tomatoes with the bacon, spinach mixture, poached eggs, and extra black pepper.

Poached Eggs with Spicy Tomato Sauce

SERVES 2 TO 4

This recipe is based on the Israeli breakfast dish shakshuka, *and the savory tomatoes and golden, runny yolks make for a filling morning meal.*

2 TABLESPOONS EXTRA-VIRGIN OLIVE OIL
1 OR 2 JALAPEÑO PEPPERS, SEEDED AND FINELY CHOPPED
1 CUP CHOPPED YELLOW ONION
3 GARLIC CLOVES, THINLY SLICED
½ TEASPOON GROUND CUMIN
1½ TEASPOONS SWEET OR SMOKED PAPRIKA
5 OR 6 BEEFSTEAK OR VINE-RIPENED TOMATOES, CHOPPED, OR 2 CUPS BOXED NO-SALT-ADDED CHOPPED TOMATOES, WITH JUICES
¼ CUP WATER
¼ TEASPOON SEA SALT
¼ TEASPOON FRESHLY GROUND BLACK PEPPER, PLUS MORE FOR GARNISH
4 EGGS
4 CUPS BABY SPINACH
3 TABLESPOONS CHOPPED FRESH FLAT-LEAF PARSLEY (OPTIONAL)

1. Heat the olive oil in a large skillet over medium-high heat. Add the jalapeños and onion and cook, stirring occasionally, until they are soft and browned, about 5 minutes.

2. Add the garlic, cumin, and paprika, and cook, stirring frequently, until fragrant, about 2 more minutes.

3. Add the tomatoes and water. Reduce the heat to medium and simmer, stirring occasionally, until the tomatoes cook down and thicken slightly, about 15 minutes. Season the tomatoes with salt and pepper.

4. Carefully crack the eggs over the sauce (or crack them into a small bowl and slide them into skillet) so that they are evenly distributed throughout the pan. Cover and cook the eggs until the yolks are just set and the whites are cooked, about 5 minutes.

5. Carefully spoon the eggs and tomato sauce over a bed of spinach and serve with extra pepper and parsley (if using).

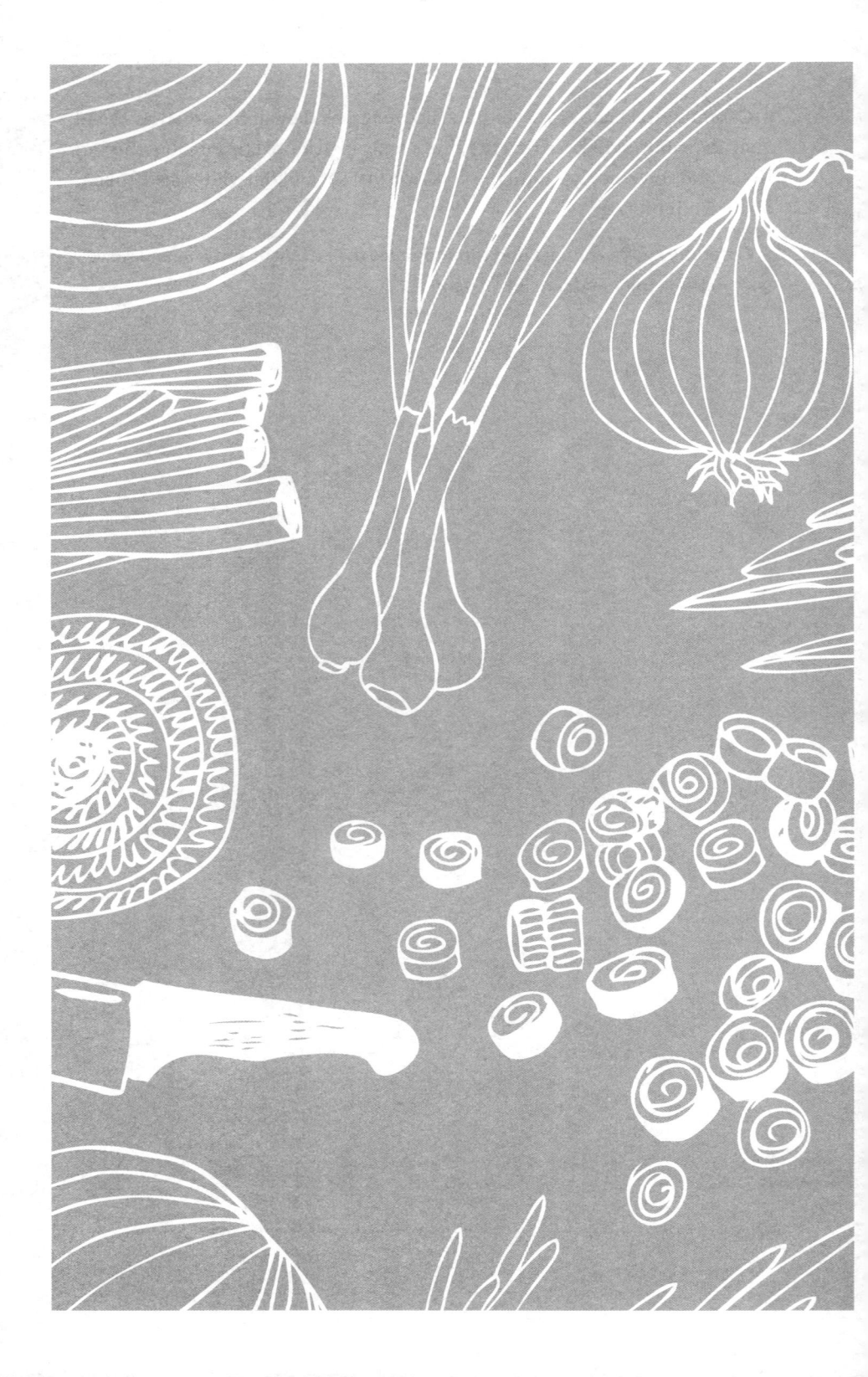

CHAPTER SEVEN

Lunch

CURRIED EGG SALAD

TUNA SALAD–STUFFED TOMATOES

GRILLED CHICKEN "CAESAR" SALAD

STEAK SALAD WITH PUMPKIN SEEDS AND CREAMY CILANTRO-LIME VINAIGRETTE

WALDORF SALAD WITH CHICKEN, APPLES, AND WALNUTS

CHICKEN "NOODLE" SOUP

CHICKEN, KALE, AND LEEK SOUP

ROASTED BUTTERNUT SQUASH AND PULLED CHICKEN SOUP

GAZPACHO WITH CRAB

SMOKED SALMON SUSHI ROLL-UPS

FRIED CAULIFLOWER "RICE" WITH SHRIMP

SALMON BURGERS WITH CARROT-CABBAGE SLAW

BUNLESS BURGERS WITH SWEET POTATO FRIES

BEEF "TACOS" WITH SALSA AND GUACAMOLE

CHILE-RUBBED CHICKEN FAJITAS WITH AVOCADO

Curried Egg Salad

SERVES 2

Homemade mayo is a great Paleo staple and comes in handy for this quick and easy, spiced-up take on a classic salad.

4 HARD-BOILED EGGS, PEELED AND CHOPPED
1 TABLESPOON DIJON MUSTARD
2 TABLESPOONS MAYONNAISE (PAGE 163)
½ TEASPOON CURRY POWDER, OR MORE, IF DESIRED
½ TEASPOON SEA SALT
2 TABLESPOONS CHOPPED FRESH CHIVES OR GREEN ONION
3 CUPS PACKED BABY SPINACH OR MIXED SPRING GREENS

1. Combine the eggs, mustard, mayonnaise, curry powder, and salt in a medium bowl and mix well.

2. Stir in the chives.

3. Serve the egg mixture over the spring greens.

Tuna Salad–Stuffed Tomatoes

SERVES 1 TO 2

Here's a great way to put tomatoes to use. If tomatoes are out of season, red bell peppers make a great substitution.

2 LARGE BEEFSTEAK, HEIRLOOM, OR VINE-RIPENED TOMATOES
1 AVOCADO, PEELED, SEEDED, AND DICED
1 (5- TO 6-OUNCE) CAN WHITE TUNA IN WATER, DRAINED AND FLAKED
2 TEASPOONS FRESH LIME JUICE
1½ TABLESPOONS AVOCADO OIL OR EXTRA-VIRGIN OLIVE OIL
½ CUP CHOPPED ARUGULA OR BABY SPINACH
1 TABLESPOON TOASTED PUMPKIN SEEDS (OPTIONAL)

1. Cut the tomatoes in half crosswise. Use a small knife to cut out the juice and pulp from each half, setting the shells aside. Chop the tomato pulp and place it in a medium bowl.

2. Add the avocado, tuna, lime juice, and oil and toss well. Add the arugula and toss again.

3. Spoon the mixture into the tomato shells and serve, topped with toasted pumpkin seeds (if using).

Grilled Chicken "Caesar" Salad

SERVES 4

Anchovies offer heart-healthful fats, but eat them in moderation because of their high sodium levels. Toasted nuts and seeds provide extra crunch in place of bready croutons.

1 TABLESPOON EXTRA-VIRGIN OLIVE OIL
4 (4- TO 6-OUNCE) BONELESS, SKINLESS CHICKEN BREASTS
1 SMALL JAR ANCHOVIES, DRAINED (OPTIONAL)
3 TABLESPOONS MAYONNAISE (PAGE 163)
2 TABLESPOONS SHERRY VINEGAR
1 GARLIC CLOVE, MINCED
¼ TEASPOON FRESHLY GROUND BLACK PEPPER
8 CUPS TORN ROMAINE LETTUCE
1 CUP DICED UNPEELED CUCUMBER
1 CUP CHERRY TOMATOES
⅓ CUP TOASTED CHOPPED WALNUTS OR PUMPKIN SEEDS

1. Heat a cast-iron grill pan over medium-high heat. Brush the oil over the chicken, and grill the chicken for 4 to 5 minutes per side or until no longer pink in the center.

2. Meanwhile, if using anchovies, place 1 or 2 drained anchovies in a small bowl and mash them with a fork. Add the mayonnaise, vinegar, garlic, and pepper and mix well.

3. Arrange the lettuce on four large plates. Divide the cucumber and tomatoes evenly among the lettuce pieces.

4. Cut the chicken crosswise into thin strips and arrange the strips over the lettuce.

5. Drizzle the anchovy dressing over the salads and top them with the nuts. Add the extra drained anchovies to the salads (if using).

Steak Salad with Pumpkin Seeds and Creamy Cilantro-Lime Vinaigrette

SERVES 4

Have extra steak on hand? Use it in this easy salad, or cook up another batch on the fly. Avocado adds a rich, creamy consistency to this dressing without the need for heavy cream.

¼ CUP EXTRA-VIRGIN OLIVE OIL
3 TABLESPOONS FRESH LIME JUICE
2 GARLIC CLOVES, MINCED
½ TEASPOON SEA SALT
½ TEASPOON HOT SAUCE OR CRUSHED RED PEPPER FLAKES
1 POUND SKIRT OR FLAT IRON STEAK
1 AVOCADO, PEELED AND SEEDED
1 CUP CILANTRO LEAVES
8 CUPS MIXED SALAD GREENS
½ CUP UNSALTED RAW OR TOASTED PUMPKIN SEEDS

1. Heat a grill or cast-iron grill pan to medium-high heat.

2. Combine the oil, lime juice, garlic, salt, and hot sauce in a small bowl and mix well.

3. Brush 3 tablespoons of the oil mixture over the steak. Grill the steak for 4 to 5 minutes per side for medium doneness.

4. Scoop half of the avocado into a blender or food processor. Add the cilantro and remaining oil mixture to the bowl and process until creamy.

5. Add the salad greens to the large bowl and toss with the dressing.

6. Dice the remaining half avocado.

7. Arrange the salad on four serving plates. Carve the steak crosswise into thin strips and arrange the strips over the salads. Top each salad with diced avocado and pumpkin seeds to serve.

Waldorf Salad with Chicken, Apples, and Walnuts

SERVES 4

Skip the cheese for extra walnuts in this classic recipe, and you'll get a double-dose of heart-healthful oils.

1 TABLESPOON WALNUT OIL
1 TABLESPOON DIJON MUSTARD
1 TABLESPOON APPLE CIDER VINEGAR
4 CUPS CHOPPED COOKED CHICKEN
1 UNPEELED RED APPLE, CHOPPED
⅓ CUP CHOPPED WALNUTS, TOASTED
4 LARGE RED LEAF OR ROMAINE LETTUCE LEAVES

1. Combine the oil, mustard, and vinegar in a medium bowl and mix well.

2. Add the chicken, apple, and walnuts, and toss until lightly coated.

3. Serve the salad on a bed of lettuce leaves.

Chicken "Noodle" Soup

SERVES 4

Just like the "real" thing but better for you, this comforting soup will warm your body and soul.

1 SMALL SPAGHETTI SQUASH (ABOUT 1 POUND)
4 CUPS BOXED NO-SALT-ADDED CHICKEN BROTH
2 SLIM CARROTS, VERY THINLY SLICED
2 CUPS CHOPPED COOKED CHICKEN (LEFTOVER OR ROTISSERIE)
3 CUPS PACKED CHOPPED KALE, SPINACH, OR SWISS CHARD LEAVES

1. Prick the squash all over with a small sharp knife. Place the squash on a paper towel in a microwave oven. Cook on high for 4 minutes.

2. Turn the squash over and continue to cook it until the squash gives when pressed gently, 4 to 5 minutes longer.

3. Allow the squash to cool for 5 minutes. While the squash is still hot, cut off and discard the stem.

4. Carefully halve the squash lengthwise (it will emit steam) and discard the seeds. Working over a bowl, scrape out the squash flesh with a fork, loosening and separating the strands.

5. Combine the broth and carrots in a large saucepan, and bring to a boil over high heat. Reduce the heat and simmer for 5 minutes.

6. Stir in the chicken and kale and simmer for 5 minutes.

7. Stir in 2 cups of the squash strands, reserving the remaining strands for another use.

8. Serve the soup hot.

Chicken, Kale, and Leek Soup

SERVES 4

This soup is a great way to get your fill of kale, and lightened-up chicken meatballs and leeks add a savory element.

1 POUND GROUND CHICKEN
1 EGG, BEATEN
2 TABLESPOONS MINCED FRESH FLAT-LEAF PARSLEY
½ TEASPOON SEA SALT
½ TEASPOON FRESHLY GROUND BLACK PEPPER
2 TABLESPOONS EXTRA-VIRGIN OLIVE OIL
1 LEEK, WHITE AND LIGHT GREEN PARTS ONLY, CHOPPED
6 CUPS CHICKEN BROTH (PAGE 158) OR BOXED NO-SALT-ADDED CHICKEN BROTH
4 CUPS CHOPPED KALE LEAVES

1. Preheat the oven to 375°F.

2. Combine the chicken, egg, parsley, salt, and pepper.

3. Roll the mixture into bite-size (¾-inch) balls and place them on a greased baking sheet. Bake the meatballs for 10 minutes.

4. Meanwhile, heat the olive oil in a large saucepan over medium heat. Add the leek and sauté for 5 minutes.

5. Add the broth and bring it to a boil. Stir in the kale, turn down the heat, and simmer for 5 minutes.

6. Stir in the cooked meatballs and simmer for another 5 minutes before serving the soup.

Roasted Butternut Squash and Pulled Chicken Soup

SERVES 4 TO 6

Butternut squash stands well on its own, but chicken adds a little extra protein. Coconut milk adds creaminess and extra taste in place of extra butter or cream, which is found in most squash soups.

1 MEDIUM TO LARGE BUTTERNUT SQUASH

2 TABLESPOONS EXTRA-VIRGIN OLIVE OIL, DIVIDED

½ CUP CHOPPED YELLOW ONION

3 CUPS CHICKEN BROTH (PAGE 158) OR BOXED NO-SALT-ADDED CHICKEN BROTH

1 CUP UNSWEETENED COCONUT MILK

¼ TEASPOON GROUND NUTMEG

¼ TEASPOON SEA SALT

¼ TEASPOON FRESHLY GROUND BLACK PEPPER

2 CUPS SHREDDED ROTISSERIE OR LEFTOVER COOKED CHICKEN

2 TO 3 TABLESPOONS UNSALTED ROASTED PISTACHIOS OR CHOPPED UNSALTED WALNUTS

1. Preheat the oven to 350°F.

2. Cut the squash in half lengthwise and scoop out the seeds. Brush the squash with 1 tablespoon of the oil and place it cut-side up on a baking sheet lined with foil. Bake the squash for 35 to 40 minutes or until very tender.

3. Heat the remaining oil in a large saucepan over medium heat. Add the onion and sauté it for 3 minutes or until tender.

4. Scoop the squash out of the skins and add it to the saucepan, mashing it with a wooden spoon.

5. Stir in the broth, coconut milk, and nutmeg. Return the saucepan to medium heat and simmer for 15 to 20 minutes.

continued ▶

Roasted Butternut Squash and Pulled Chicken Soup *continued* ▶

6. Transfer the soup to a blender and process until smooth; then return the soup to the saucepan.

7. Season the soup with salt and pepper. Stir in chicken and cook until it is heated through.

8. Serve the soup with pistachios or walnuts.

Gazpacho with Crab

SERVES 2

Typically enjoyed during the summer when fresh produce is available, gazpacho may be eaten year-round using boxed tomatoes or those jarred during the summer months.

8 PLUM TOMATOES, PLUS THEIR JUICES, OR 2 CUPS BOXED NO-SALT-ADDED WHOLE TOMATOES AND JUICES
1 YELLOW OR RED BELL PEPPER, ROUGHLY CHOPPED
1 SMALL CUCUMBER, ROUGHLY CHOPPED
1 JALAPEÑO PEPPER, SEEDED
⅓ CUP ROUGHLY CHOPPED RED ONION
⅓ CUP EXTRA-VIRGIN OLIVE OR AVOCADO OIL
1 TABLESPOON BALSAMIC OR RED WINE VINEGAR
1 AVOCADO
2 CUPS FRESH LUMP CRABMEAT, SHREDDED

1. Add the tomatoes, bell pepper, cucumber, jalapeño, red onion, oil, and vinegar to a blender or food processor and process until smooth. Refrigerate the mixture for at least 2 hours.

2. Just before serving, peel, seed, and dice the avocado.

3. Ladle the gazpacho into shallow bowls and top each with the avocado and crabmeat.

Smoked Salmon Sushi Roll-Ups

SERVES 2

Cucumbers and carrots stand in as antioxidant-rich substitutes for plain white rice in this sushi-like recipe. This is great for a quick, no-cook lunch.

1 AVOCADO, PEELED, SEEDED, AND DICED
2 TABLESPOONS FINELY DICED CUCUMBER
2 TABLESPOONS THINLY SLICED GREEN ONIONS
2 TEASPOONS GRATED FRESH GINGER
1 TEASPOON WASABI PASTE (OPTIONAL)
4 OUNCES SMOKED WILD-CAUGHT SALMON SLICES
2 NORI SHEETS, SOFTENED FOR 5 MINUTES IN WARM WATER
1 CARROT, CUT INTO MATCHSTICK PIECES
½ CUCUMBER, CUT INTO MATCHSTICK PIECES
3 TABLESPOONS GLUTEN-FREE SOY SAUCE, SUCH AS TAMARI OR BRAGG LIQUID AMINOS
2 TEASPOONS TOASTED SESAME OIL

1. Combine the avocado, cucumber, green onions, ginger, and wasabi paste (if using) in a medium bowl and mix well.

2. Divide the salmon between the nori sheets, layering over one half of the sheet.

3. Spread the avocado mixture over the other half of the sheet. Top the avocado mixture with the carrots and cucumbers and roll it up, working from the longer side, into a long spiral.

4. Cut each roll crosswise into 2 smaller rolls. Serve the rolls with combined soy sauce and sesame oil for dipping.

Fried Cauliflower "Rice" with Shrimp

SERVES 4

Craving a little rice? This cauliflower version satisfies just as much with far more nutritional benefits than the calorie-dense, nutrient-poor alternative.

1 HEAD CAULIFLOWER, STEMS REMOVED
2 TABLESPOONS COCONUT OIL
1 RED BELL PEPPER, DICED
1 CUP SLICED SNOW PEAS
1 CARROT, PEELED AND CUT INTO MATCHSTICK PIECES
2 CUPS SHRIMP, PEELED AND DEVEINED
1 EGG, BEATEN
1 TABLESPOON GLUTEN-FREE SOY SAUCE, SUCH AS TAMARI OR BRAGG LIQUID AMINOS
½ TABLESPOON TOASTED SESAME OIL
2 GREEN ONIONS, SLICED
1 TEASPOON RED PEPPER FLAKES (OPTIONAL)
3 TABLESPOONS SESAME SEEDS (OPTIONAL)
1 CUP CHOPPED FRESH CILANTRO (OPTIONAL)

1. Place the cauliflower in a food processor or blender, and pulse until it is the consistency of rice.

2. In a large wok or skillet, heat the oil over medium-high heat. Add the bell pepper, peas, and carrot and cook until the vegetables beginning to soften, 3 to 4 minutes.

3. Add the shrimp and cook until it is opaque.

4. Stir in the egg until it is cooked, about 2 minutes.

5. Add the cauliflower rice, tamari, sesame oil, green onions, and red pepper flakes (if using). Toss until heated through.

6. Serve this dish with sesame seeds and cilantro (if using).

Salmon Burgers with Carrot-Cabbage Slaw

SERVES 4

Leftover salmon gets put to great use in this easy, omega-3-rich recipe. If buying the canned version, choose wild-caught Alaskan salmon for the most sustainable purchase. Wrap and freeze any leftover burgers, and reheat them in a skillet or in the oven whenever you need a quick meal.

FOR THE SLAW:
2 CUPS SHREDDED RED CABBAGE
1 CARROT, SHREDDED
3 TABLESPOONS EXTRA-VIRGIN OLIVE OIL
1 TABLESPOON APPLE CIDER VINEGAR
2 TEASPOONS DIJON MUSTARD
¼ TEASPOON FRESHLY GROUND BLACK PEPPER

FOR THE SALMON BURGERS:
1¾ CUPS FLAKED COOKED FRESH SALMON OR 1 TO 2 CANS SALMON (14.5 OUNCES TOTAL), SKIN AND BONES DISCARDED
½ CUP ALMOND MEAL
1 EGG
2 TABLESPOONS FINELY CHOPPED FRESH CILANTRO, PLUS MORE FOR GARNISH
2 TABLESPOONS FINELY CHOPPED YELLOW ONION
¼ TEASPOON SEA SALT
¼ TEASPOON FRESHLY GROUND BLACK PEPPER
2 TABLESPOONS EXTRA-VIRGIN OLIVE OIL
LIME OR LEMON WEDGES, FOR GARNISH

To make the slaw:

Toss together all the ingredients. Cover and refrigerate the slaw until it's ready to be used.

To make the salmon burgers:

1. Combine the salmon, almond meal, egg, cilantro, onion, salt, and pepper, mixing well.

2. Shape the mixture into 4 patties, each about ½ inch thick.

3. Heat the oil in a large nonstick skillet over medium heat until hot. Add the patties and cook for 4 minutes per side or until golden brown.

4. Serve the salmon burgers topped with the slaw and garnished with the lime or lemon wedges.

Bunless Burgers with Sweet Potato Fries

SERVES 4

You won't miss the bun or the fries with this tastier version. Sweet potatoes pack more vitamins and satisfy even more than their white tubular siblings. Freeze leftover cooked or uncooked burger patties for quick lunches and dinners.

2 MEDIUM SWEET POTATOES
2 TABLESPOONS EXTRA-VIRGIN OLIVE OR MELTED COCONUT OIL
1 POUND GROUND BEEF CHUCK OR BISON
½ TEASPOON SEA SALT
1 TEASPOON FRESHLY GROUND BLACK PEPPER
¼ CUP DIJON MUSTARD
4 LARGE BIBB LETTUCE LEAVES (OPTIONAL)

1. Preheat the oven to 425°F.

2. Cut each sweet potato in half lengthwise; then cut each half into 4 wedges and place them in a large bowl. Add the oil and toss well.

3. Arrange the sweet potatoes on a large rimmed baking sheet in one layer and bake for 10 minutes.

4. Meanwhile, combine the meat with ¼ teaspoon of the salt and ½ teaspoon of the pepper. Mix the meat lightly and form it into four ½-inch-thick patties.

5. Remove the potatoes from the oven and turn them over with a large spatula. Sprinkle the remaining ¼ teaspoon of salt and ½ teaspoon of pepper evenly over the potatoes. Return them to the oven and bake for 10 to 12 minutes or until the potatoes are tender.

6. Cook the patties in a large nonstick skillet over medium heat for 5 to 6 minutes per side or until barely pink in the center. (Patties may also be cooked on a grill over medium-high heat.)

7. Top the burgers with mustard and serve them with the sweet potato fries. Wrap the burgers in lettuce leaves before serving (if using).

Beef "Tacos" with Salsa and Guacamole

SERVES 4

No need for tortillas—lettuce leaves pack a stronger nutritional punch. Ground turkey, chicken, or even leftover chorizo may easily be substituted for the beef in this recipe, if desired.

1 POUND GROUND BEEF
1 TEASPOON GROUND CUMIN
½ TEASPOON CAYENNE PEPPER
¼ TEASPOON SEA SALT
1 TO 2 TABLESPOONS EXTRA-VIRGIN OLIVE OR AVOCADO OIL
1 BUNCH FRESH CILANTRO LEAVES, CHOPPED
1 RED ONION, DICED
2 PEELED CARROTS OR JICAMA, SHAVED
8 LARGE BIBB OR ROMAINE LETTUCE LEAVES
½ CUP NO-SUGAR-ADDED NATURAL SALSA OR ROASTED TOMATO SALSA (PAGE 166)
½ CUP GUACAMOLE (PAGE 165) OR AVOCADO SLICES

1. Season the beef with the cumin, cayenne, and salt.

2. Heat the oil in a large skillet over medium-high heat. Cook the beef until it is browned, about 5 minutes, stirring occasionally.

3. Toss the beef with the cilantro, onion, and carrots.

4. Serve the tacos on lettuce leaves with salsa and guacamole or avocado slices.

Chile-Rubbed Chicken Fajitas with Avocado

SERVES 4

Large lettuce leaves make for a great sub-in for tortillas in Paleo "taco" and fajita recipes, like this one. Make your own salt-free ancho chili powder by grinding dried ancho chiles in a food processor blender.

1 POUND SKINLESS BONELESS CHICKEN BREAST, CUT CROSSWISE INTO ½-INCH-THICK STRIPS
2 TEASPOONS ANCHO CHILI POWDER OR CAYENNE PEPPER
1 TEASPOON GROUND CUMIN
¼ TEASPOON SEA SALT
3 TABLESPOONS EXTRA-VIRGIN OLIVE OIL
1 RED BELL PEPPER, THINLY SLICED
1 GREEN BELL PEPPER, THINLY SLICED
1 YELLOW ONION, THINLY SLICED
½ CUP ROASTED TOMATO SALSA (PAGE 166) OR NO-SUGAR-ADDED SALSA
8 LARGE BOSTON OR ROMAINE LETTUCE LEAVES
1 AVOCADO, PEELED, SEEDED, AND SLICED
LIME WEDGES, FOR GARNISH

1. Toss the chicken with the chili powder, cumin, and salt.

2. Heat the oil in a large skillet over medium-high heat. Add the bell peppers and onion and stir-fry for 4 minutes.

3. Add the chicken strips and stir-fry them until they are browned, about 4 minutes.

4. Add the salsa and simmer until the chicken is cooked through, about 2 minutes.

5. Serve the fajitas in lettuce leaves topped with avocado and garnished with lime wedges.

CHAPTER EIGHT

Dinner

ASPARAGUS LEEK "RISOTTO" WITH SCALLOPS

CHICKEN VESUVIO WITH SWEET POTATOES

SPANISH CHICKEN WITH ROMESCO SAUCE

MUSTARD-CRUSTED CHICKEN THIGHS AND GARLICKY GREENS

HERBED TURKEY MEATBALLS WITH SPAGHETTI SQUASH

SPICY ITALIAN FISH STEW WITH FENNEL

HALIBUT STEAKS WITH SALSA VERDE

CHARD-WRAPPED ARCTIC CHAR WITH BALSAMIC GLAZE

LEMON-POACHED SALMON WITH ROASTED BALSAMIC-GLAZED KALE AND CHERRY TOMATOES

LAMB KEBABS WITH PARSLEY-MINT SAUCE

CUBAN PULLED PORK

MAPLE-GLAZED PORK CHOPS WITH ROASTED BRUSSELS SPROUTS, BACON, AND WALNUTS

STIR-FRIED PORK WITH BROCCOLI AND RED PEPPER

TEXAS-STYLE BEEF CHILI

CLASSIC BEEF STEW WITH SWEET POTATOES

KOREAN BARBECUE BEEF LETTUCE WRAPS

ARGENTINEAN SKIRT STEAK WITH CHIMICHURRI

STANDING RIB ROAST WITH MUSTARD-HORSERADISH SAUCE

TRI-COLORED EGGPLANT "LASAGNA" WITH SAUSAGE

ITALIAN SAUSAGE–STUFFED PEPPERS

Asparagus Leek "Risotto" with Scallops

SERVES 4

This Paleo-friendly "risotto" uses cauliflower instead of rice, which pairs great with savory leeks and meaty scallops. Store leftover risotto in the refrigerator for three days, or in the freezer for up to a month, and pair it with other proteins like eggs and cooked chicken.

1 SMALL HEAD CAULIFLOWER
1 CUP 1-INCH PIECES FRESH ASPARAGUS
2 CUPS BOXED NO-SALT-ADDED VEGETABLE BROTH OR HOMEMADE VEGETABLE BROTH (SEE CHICKEN BROTH RECIPE, PAGE 158)
1 TABLESPOON EXTRA-VIRGIN OLIVE OIL
1½ POUNDS SCALLOPS
¼ TEASPOON SEA SALT
¼ TEASPOON FRESHLY GROUND BLACK PEPPER
½ CUP DICED LEEKS, WHITE AND LIGHT GREEN PARTS ONLY
¼ CUP FRESH LEMON JUICE
CHOPPED FRESH FLAT-LEAF PARSLEY (OPTIONAL)

1. Cut the cauliflower into large florets, saving the tough stems for another use. In batches, pulse the cauliflower in a food processor until it is chopped and about the size of rice.

2. Combine the asparagus and vegetable broth in a medium saucepan. Bring the broth to a boil over high heat. Reduce the heat and simmer the asparagus until it is crisp-tender, 3 to 4 minutes. Use a slotted spoon to transfer asparagus to a bowl, and set it aside. Keep the broth at a simmer in the saucepan.

3. In a separate heavy skillet, heat the oil over medium-high heat. Season the scallops with salt and pepper and add them to the skillet. Cook the scallops for 3 minutes on each side or until they are browned and just cooked through in the center. Remove the scallops and set them aside.

4. In the same skillet, add the leeks and sauté them for 3 minutes.

5. Stir in the lemon juice and cook for 2 minutes.

6. Add the cauliflower and ¼ cup of the broth. Sauté the vegetables until the broth is absorbed.

7. Continue adding ¼ cupfuls of broth at a time, cooking and stirring until the broth is absorbed each time.

8. When all of broth is absorbed, stir in the asparagus and heat through.

9. Serve the risotto topped with the scallops and garnished with parsley (if using).

Chicken Vesuvio with Sweet Potatoes

SERVES 4

This classic Italian dish never fails, and it tastes just as great if not better with beta-carotene-rich sweet potatoes. Save the bones from the chicken (and ask for the back and neck bones if purchasing the chicken from a butcher) to make homemade Chicken Broth (page 158).

⅓ CUP EXTRA-VIRGIN OLIVE OIL, PLUS MORE FOR THE PAN
1 WHOLE FRESH CHICKEN (ABOUT 3½ POUNDS), QUARTERED
2 LARGE SWEET POTATOES, CUT LENGTHWISE INTO 6 WEDGES
¼ CUP FRESH LEMON JUICE
3 TO 4 GARLIC CLOVES, MINCED
PINCH OF SEA SALT
PINCH OF FRESHLY GROUND BLACK PEPPER
1 TEASPOON GRATED LEMON PEEL
1 TEASPOON DRIED OR 1 TABLESPOON CHOPPED FRESH ROSEMARY OR OREGANO

1. Preheat the oven to 375°F.

2. Oil a very large shallow roasting pan or two jelly roll pans. Place the chicken quarters in the center of the pan; place the potato wedges peel-side down around chicken.

3. Combine ⅓ cup of the oil, lemon juice, and garlic; pour the mixture evenly over the chicken and potatoes.

4. Sprinkle the chicken and potatoes liberally with salt and freshly ground black pepper; then bake the chicken and potatoes for 30 minutes.

5. Baste the chicken and potatoes with the pan juices. Sprinkle the lemon peel and rosemary over the chicken.

6. Continue baking the chicken and potatoes for another 30 to 40 minutes or until the chicken is cooked through and the potatoes are tender. Serve hot.

Spanish Chicken with Romesco Sauce

SERVES 4

Looking to add a bit of spice to your chicken dinner? Romesco sauce will do just that with its flavorful blend of hazelnuts, cloves, and red pepper flakes.

4 BONE-IN CHICKEN BREASTS
2 TABLESPOONS EXTRA-VIRGIN OLIVE OIL
2 TEASPOONS PAPRIKA OR SMOKED PAPRIKA
½ TEASPOON SEA SALT
½ TEASPOON FRESHLY GROUND BLACK PEPPER
1 (7- TO 8-OUNCE) JAR ROASTED RED PEPPERS, DRAINED AND RINSED
2 TABLESPOONS UNSALTED RAW OR BLANCHED ALMONDS
2 TABLESPOONS UNSALTED ROASTED HAZELNUTS
1 GARLIC CLOVE
¼ TEASPOON RED PEPPER FLAKES
1 TABLESPOON RED WINE VINEGAR

1. Preheat the oven to 375°F.

2. Place the chicken on a rimmed baking sheet. Brush 1 tablespoon of the oil over the chicken.

3. Combine the paprika, salt, and pepper and sprinkle it over the chicken.

4. Bake the chicken for 40 to 50 minutes or until the internal temperature reaches 165°F.

5. Meanwhile, for the sauce, add the roasted red peppers, almonds, hazelnuts, garlic, pepper flakes, vinegar, and remaining 1 tablespoon of oil to a blender or food processor. Process until smooth.

6. Serve the chicken with the sauce.

Mustard-Crusted Chicken Thighs and Garlicky Greens

SERVES 4

This hands-off dish is great for weeknight meals and a perfect way to use extra chicken thighs you might have in your freezer.

4 LARGE OR 8 SMALL BONE-IN CHICKEN THIGHS
¼ CUP DIJON MUSTARD
¼ TEASPOON SEA SALT
¼ TEASPOON FRESHLY GROUND BLACK PEPPER
1 TEASPOON SMOKED PAPRIKA
1 TABLESPOON EXTRA-VIRGIN OLIVE OIL
1 LARGE BUNCH MUSTARD GREENS, COLLARD GREENS, OR SWISS CHARD, TOUGH STEMS DISCARDED AND LEAVES CHOPPED
3 GARLIC CLOVES, MINCED

1. Preheat the oven to 375°F.

2. Arrange the chicken in a shallow roasting pan. Spread the mustard evenly over the chicken.

3. In a small bowl, combine the salt, pepper, and paprika. Sprinkle the seasoning blend over the chicken.

4. Bake the chicken for 45 to 55 minutes or until an internal meat thermometer reads 165°F and the juices run clear.

5. While the chicken is roasting, heat the oil in large saucepan over medium-high heat. Add the greens and garlic. Cover and cook the greens for 2 minutes or until they are wilted.

6. Uncover the greens and turn them with tongs until they are evenly wilted.

7. Remove the chicken from the oven and serve it with the greens.

Herbed Turkey Meatballs with Spaghetti Squash

SERVES 4 TO 6

Packed with herbs, these turkey meatballs are bursting with flavor, while spaghetti squash stands in even better for the flour version. For a heartier version, swap ground turkey for ground beef, bison, or ground pork.

1 POUND GROUND TURKEY

2 TABLESPOONS CHOPPED FRESH BASIL, PLUS ½ CUP FOR GARNISH

2 TABLESPOONS CHOPPED FRESH FLAT-LEAF PARSLEY

1 TEASPOON DRIED OREGANO

½ TEASPOON SEA SALT

½ TEASPOON FRESHLY GROUND BLACK PEPPER

2 TABLESPOONS EXTRA-VIRGIN OLIVE OIL

2 CUPS TOMATO SAUCE (PAGE 157) OR BOXED NO-SUGAR-ADDED TOMATO SAUCE

1 (3- TO 3¼-POUND) SPAGHETTI SQUASH

1. Combine the turkey, 2 tablespoons of the basil, parsley, oregano, salt, and pepper in a mixing bowl and mix well. Using wet hands, shape the mixture into 2-inch balls.

2. Heat 1 tablespoon of oil in a large skillet over medium-high heat. Add the meatballs and cook them until they are browned, about 5 minutes, turning as needed.

3. Pour the Tomato Sauce into the skillet and bring it to a simmer. Cover the skillet, reduce the heat to medium-low, and cook until the meatballs are no longer pink in the center.

4. Meanwhile, prick the squash all over with a small sharp knife. Place it on a paper towel or microwave-safe plate in a microwave oven. Cook the squash on high for 8 minutes.

continued ▶

Herbed Turkey Meatballs with Spaghetti Squash *continued* ▶

5. Turn the squash over and continue to cook it until the squash gives when pressed gently, 5 to 7 minutes, depending on the size of the squash.

6. Allow the squash to cool for 5 minutes. While squash is still hot, cut off and discard the stem.

7. Carefully halve the squash lengthwise (it will emit steam) and discard the seeds. Working over a bowl, scrape out the squash flesh with a fork, loosening and separating strands. Toss the squash strands in the remaining 1 tablespoon of olive oil.

8. Arrange squash strands on four serving plates. Serve the meatballs and sauce over the squash, and garnish it with ½ cup of basil.

Spicy Italian Fish Stew with Fennel

SERVES 4

This Italian fish stew gets stepped up a notch with herbaceous fennel and spicy red pepper flakes.

1 FENNEL BULB WITH FRONDS
2 TABLESPOONS EXTRA-VIRGIN OLIVE OIL
3 GARLIC CLOVES, MINCED
2 CUPS FRESH OR BOXED NO-SALT-ADDED CHOPPED TOMATOES, WITH JUICES
½ CUP FILTERED WATER
¼ TEASPOON DRIED OREGANO
½ TEASPOON RED PEPPER FLAKES
1 POUND TILAPIA OR OTHER WHITEFISH FILLETS, CUT INTO 1-INCH PIECES

1. Slice off the fronds from the fennel bulb, chop them finely, and set them aside.

2. Cut the fennel bulb in half. Remove and discard the core and thinly slice the bulb.

3. Heat the oil in a large Dutch oven or heavy-bottomed pot over medium-high heat. Add the chopped fennel bulb and cook it until it is softened, about 2 minutes.

4. Add the garlic and cook for 1 minute, or until the garlic is fragrant.

5. Add the tomatoes, water, oregano, and red pepper flakes and simmer for 5 minutes.

6. Add the fish, cover, and simmer the ingredients for 4 to 5 minutes or until the fish is cooked through.

7. Serve the stew topped with the fennel fronds.

Halibut Steaks with Salsa Verde

SERVES 4

This tasty green salsa bumps up halibut's mild flavor without the need for extra salt. Serve it with green beans or lightly sautéed or steamed spinach.

4 (6- TO 8-OUNCE) HALIBUT STEAKS, SKIN REMOVED
¼ TEASPOON SEA SALT
¼ TEASPOON FRESHLY GROUND BLACK PEPPER
4 FRESH TOMATILLOS
½ CUP FRESH LIME JUICE
1 TO 2 CUPS FRESH CILANTRO, STEMS DISCARDED, PLUS MORE FOR GARNISH
1 SERRANO PEPPER, SEEDED AND FINELY CHOPPED
1 AVOCADO, PEELED, SEEDED, AND DICED

1. Preheat the broiler to high heat.

2. Place the halibut steaks on a foil-lined sheet tray and season them with salt and pepper.

3. In a small saucepan, boil the tomatillos in water for 5 minutes or until almost tender. Drain and allow the tomatillos to cool before transferring them to a blender or food processor.

4. Add the lime juice, cilantro, serrano pepper, and avocado to the blender. Pulse until the mixture is just slightly chunky.

5. Broil the halibut steaks until they are browned on top and opaque in the center, 6 to 8 minutes.

6. Serve the halibut steaks with the salsa verde and extra chopped cilantro.

Chard-Wrapped Arctic Char with Balsamic Glaze

SERVES 4

You'll easily get your daily dose of omega-3s with this light and nutritious dinner. If arctic char is unavailable, substitute with any other meaty fish, including salmon or whitefish like cod or halibut.

½ CUP BALSAMIC VINEGAR
4 LARGE SWISS OR RAINBOW CHARD LEAVES
4 (6-OUNCE) ARCTIC CHAR FILLETS
¼ TEASPOON SEA SALT
¼ TEASPOON FRESHLY GROUND BLACK PEPPER
2 TABLESPOONS EXTRA-VIRGIN OLIVE OIL

1. In a small saucepot, heat the vinegar over medium-high heat. Boil the vinegar until it is reduced by half and slightly thickened, being careful not to burn it. Pour the vinegar immediately into a separate ceramic or glass bowl and set it aside.

2. Meanwhile, slice off the chard leaves, leaving the stems. Chop the stems into 1-inch-thick pieces and set them aside.

3. Add about 1 inch of water to a large skillet and bring it to a simmer over medium-high heat. Add the chard leaves, cover, and steam until the leaves are just wilted, 1 to 2 minutes. Blot the leaves with a paper towel and set them aside. Wipe out the skillet.

4. Season the fish with salt and pepper. Wrap 1 leaf around each fillet, enclosing as much of the fillet as possible.

5. Heat the oil in a large skillet over medium-high heat. Add the chard stem pieces and cook until they are tender, about 3 minutes.

6. Push the stems to the edges of the pan and add the fillets. Cook the fillets for 3 minutes per side or until the fish are opaque.

7. Serve the fillets with a drizzle of balsamic glaze.

Lemon-Poached Salmon with Roasted Balsamic-Glazed Kale and Cherry Tomatoes

SERVES 4

Poaching salmon in liquid preserves the healthful fat and other nutrients of the fish, while the lemon juice has powerful detox and anti-inflammation effects. Leftover salmon may be flaked and made into salmon burgers (page 102).

- 4 (4- TO 6-OUNCE) SALMON FILLETS, SKIN REMOVED
- ½ TEASPOON SEA SALT
- ½ TEASPOON FRESHLY GROUND BLACK PEPPER
- 2 TABLESPOONS BALSAMIC VINEGAR
- 2 TEASPOONS CHOPPED FRESH THYME
- 2 TABLESPOONS EXTRA-VIRGIN OLIVE OIL
- 1 PINT CHERRY TOMATOES, HALVED
- 1 BUNCH KALE, RIBS REMOVED AND ROUGHLY CHOPPED
- 1 TABLESPOON MINCED GARLIC
- ¼ CUP FRESH LEMON JUICE
- 1 CUP FILTERED WATER

1. Preheat the oven to 400°F.

2. Spray a rimmed baking sheet with cooking spray or line it with foil.

3. Season the salmon with ¼ teaspoon each of the salt and pepper.

4. In a small bowl, whisk together the vinegar, thyme, 1 tablespoon of the oil, and the remaining ¼ teaspoon each of salt and pepper.

5. Toss the tomatoes and kale with the dressing and spread the mixture onto the baking sheet.

6. Roast the tomatoes and kale for 10 minutes, or until the tomatoes are tender and the kale is just wilted and slightly browned around the edges.

7. Meanwhile, in a large skillet, heat the remaining 1 tablespoon of oil over medium-high heat. Cook the garlic until fragrant, about 1 minute.

8. Add lemon juice and water, stirring once; then reduce the heat to a simmer and add the salmon fillets. Cover and cook the salmon for 6 to 8 minutes, or until the salmon is opaque in the center and flakes easily with a fork.

9. Remove the salmon from the pan and set aside.

10. Boil the remaining liquid until it is reduced by half.

11. Spoon the sauce over the salmon and serve it alongside the roasted kale and cherry tomatoes.

Lamb Kebabs with Parsley-Mint Sauce

SERVES 4

Kebabs are an easy Paleo meal, and the variations are endless. Lamb may easily be swapped out for stew beef chunks or chicken breast pieces.

FOR THE SAUCE:

¼ CUP PACKED CHOPPED FRESH MINT LEAVES
¼ CUP PACKED CHOPPED FRESH FLAT-LEAF PARSLEY LEAVES
2 TABLESPOONS EXTRA-VIRGIN OLIVE OIL
2 TEASPOONS FRESH LEMON JUICE
2 GARLIC CLOVES, MINCED

FOR THE KEBABS:

2 TABLESPOONS FRESH LEMON JUICE
1 TEASPOON EXTRA-VIRGIN OLIVE OIL
½ TEASPOON SEA SALT
¼ TEASPOON CRUSHED RED PEPPER FLAKES
¼ TEASPOON FRESHLY GROUND BLACK PEPPER
2 GARLIC CLOVES, MINCED
1 POUND BONELESS LEG OF LAMB, CUT INTO 1-INCH PIECES

To make the sauce:

In a small bowl, combine all the ingredients and mix well. Set the sauce aside.

To make the kebabs:

1. In a medium bowl, combine the lemon juice, oil, salt, pepper flakes, black pepper, and garlic and mix well.

2. Add the lamb and toss well.

3. Let the lamb stand for 15 minutes, or cover and refrigerate it for up to 4 hours.

4. Prepare a grill or cast-iron skillet to medium-high heat.

5. Drain the lamb, reserving the marinade.

6. Thread the lamb pieces onto metal skewers and grill them for 5 minutes, brushing them with the reserved marinade. Turn the kebabs and continue grilling them for 4 to 5 more minutes or until the lamb is pink in center.

7. Serve the kebabs with the sauce.

Cuban Pulled Pork

SERVES 6

No need for a bun—this savory dinner tastes great on its own or served with large lettuce leaves for wraps. This recipe also shows why it's convenient to save bacon drippings in the refrigerator.

2 TEASPOONS SEA SALT
2 TEASPOONS PAPRIKA OR SMOKED PAPRIKA
2 TEASPOONS GROUND CUMIN
1 TEASPOON CRUSHED RED PEPPER FLAKES
2½ POUNDS BONELESS PORK SHOULDER ROAST, TRIMMED
2 TABLESPOONS RESERVED BACON DRIPPINGS OR EXTRA-VIRGIN OLIVE OIL
½ CUP FRESH LIME JUICE
½ CUP FRESH LEMON JUICE
2 CUPS CHOPPED RED ONION
10 GARLIC CLOVES, CRUSHED
½ CUP CHOPPED FRESH CILANTRO
MIXED SPRING GREENS OR LARGE BIBB LETTUCE LEAVES (OPTIONAL)
AVOCADO, PEELED, PITTED, AND SLICED (OPTIONAL)

1. Preheat the oven to 350°F.

2. Combine the salt, paprika, cumin, and pepper flakes, and rub the mixture over the entire surface of the pork roast.

3. Heat the bacon drippings in a large Dutch oven over medium heat.

4. Add the roast and brown it well on both sides, about 10 minutes total.

5. Turn off the heat and pour the lime and lemon juices over the roast. Spoon the onion and garlic around roast.

6. Cover and bake the roast for 2 to 2½ hours or until the meat is fork tender.

7. Uncover the pan and use two forks to pull the meat into shreds, mixing it with the sauce in pan. Stir in the cilantro.

8. Serve the pulled pork over a bed of greens or with lettuce wraps and avocado (if using).

Maple-Glazed Pork Chops with Roasted Brussels Sprouts, Bacon, and Walnuts

SERVES 4 TO 6

Pork chops are easy to cook, delicious, and help mix things up when it comes to selecting proteins. A little maple syrup balances out the more savory bacon and nut flavors.

⅓ CUP GRADE B PURE MAPLE SYRUP
¼ CUP APPLE CIDER VINEGAR
¼ TEASPOON SEA SALT
¼ TEASPOON FRESHLY GROUND BLACK PEPPER
4 LARGE PORK CHOPS
1 TO 1½ POUNDS BRUSSELS SPROUTS, DAMAGED OUTER LEAVES REMOVED AND HALVED LENGTHWISE
1 TABLESPOON EXTRA-VIRGIN OLIVE OIL
2 OUNCES THICK-CUT NITRATE-FREE BACON, SLICED INTO ¾-INCH CUBES
½ CUP CHOPPED UNSALTED WALNUTS

1. Preheat the oven to 375°F.

2. In a small bowl, combine the maple syrup, vinegar, salt, and pepper. Brush the pork chops with the mixture to coat it on both sides and set it aside.

3. Toss the Brussels sprouts with the olive oil and roast them for 20 to 30 minutes or until they are browned and tender. Remove the Brussels sprouts from the oven and set them aside.

4. In a large skillet over medium heat, cook the bacon and walnuts until the bacon releases its fat and the walnuts are toasted, about 4 minutes. Using a slotted spoon, transfer the bacon and walnuts to a paper towel–lined plate.

5. Add the pork chops to the same skillet and cook them until they are browned, about 3 minutes per side.

6. Toss Brussels sprouts with the bacon-walnut mixture and serve with the pork chops.

Stir-Fried Pork with Broccoli and Red Pepper

SERVES 4

This Chinese-inspired dish works just as well with beef, if desired. Leftovers will keep in the refrigerator up to three days.

1 POUND PORK TENDERLOIN
¼ CUP GLUTEN-FREE SOY SAUCE, SUCH AS TAMARI OR BRAGG LIQUID AMINOS
2 TABLESPOONS RAW HONEY, GRADE B PURE MAPLE SYRUP, OR AGAVE NECTAR
½ TEASPOON CRUSHED RED PEPPER FLAKES
2 TABLESPOONS COCONUT OIL
2 CUPS BROCCOLI FLORETS
1 RED BELL PEPPER, CUT INTO SHORT, THIN STRIPS
2 GREEN ONIONS, SLICED
⅓ CUP CHOPPED UNSALTED TOASTED ALMONDS (OPTIONAL)

1. Cut the tenderloin crosswise into thin slices; then cut each slice in half and set aside.

2. Combine the soy sauce, honey, and pepper flakes and set aside.

3. Heat the oil in a large skillet or wok over medium-high heat. Add the broccoli and bell pepper strips and stir-fry for 4 minutes.

4. Add the pork and stir-fry the mixture for another 2 minutes.

5. Add the soy sauce mixture and green onions. Stir-fry for 3 to 4 minutes or until the vegetables are crisp-tender and the sauce thickens.

6. Serve hot, topped with almonds (if using).

Texas-Style Beef Chili

SERVES 4

Texans are known for their beanless chili, which makes for a perfect Paleo meal. Freeze leftover chili in individual batches for quick lunches and dinners.

1 POUND GROUND BEEF CHUCK
1 YELLOW ONION, CHOPPED
3 GARLIC CLOVES, MINCED
2 TEASPOONS CAYENNE POWDER
2 TEASPOONS GROUND CUMIN
2 CUPS FRESH OR BOXED NO-SALT-ADDED DICED OR CRUSHED TOMATOES, WITH JUICES
1 TO 2 JALAPEÑO OR SERRANO PEPPERS, SEEDED AND FINELY CHOPPED
1 GREEN BELL PEPPER, DICED
1 RED OR YELLOW BELL PEPPER, DICED
½ CUP CHOPPED FRESH CILANTRO
1 AVOCADO, PEELED, SEEDED, AND DICED

1. Crumble the beef into a large saucepan and place it over medium heat. Cook it for 5 minutes, stirring frequently.

2. Add the onion, garlic, cayenne, and cumin. Continue cooking for 5 minutes, stirring frequently.

3. Stir in the tomatoes with juices and peppers. Bring the mixture to a simmer, and cook, uncovered, for 20 to 25 minutes or until the peppers are tender.

4. Ladle the chili into four shallow bowls, and top with the cilantro and avocado.

Classic Beef Stew with Sweet Potatoes

SERVES 4

This classic recipe swaps out white potatoes for their more nutritious sweet siblings.

1 TABLESPOON EXTRA-VIRGIN OLIVE OIL
1¼ POUNDS BEEF STEW MEAT
2 TEASPOONS DRIED THYME LEAVES
½ TEASPOON SEA SALT
½ TEASPOON FRESHLY GROUND BLACK PEPPER
¼ TEASPOON GROUND CINNAMON
¼ TEASPOON CAYENNE PEPPER
1 YELLOW ONION, COARSELY CHOPPED
4 GARLIC CLOVES, MINCED
1½ CUPS BOXED NO-SALT-ADDED BEEF BROTH OR HOMEMADE VEGETABLE BROTH (SEE CHICKEN BROTH RECIPE, PAGE 158)
2 CUPS FRESH OR BOXED NO-SALT-ADDED DICED TOMATOES WITH JUICES
6 CARROTS, THICKLY SLICED
2 LARGE SWEET POTATOES, PEELED AND CUT INTO 1-INCH CHUNKS
CHOPPED FRESH FLAT-LEAF PARSLEY OR THYME (OPTIONAL)

1. Heat the oil in a large Dutch oven over medium heat and add the meat.

2. Sprinkle the thyme, salt, pepper, cinnamon, and cayenne pepper over the meat and toss with two wooden spoons to coat. Cook until the meat is browned on all sides, turning once, about 7 to 8 minutes.

3. Stir in the onion and garlic and cook for 5 minutes.

4. Stir in the broth and tomatoes and bring to a boil over high heat. Reduce the heat and simmer, uncovered, for 40 minutes.

5. Stir in the carrots and sweet potatoes. Continue to simmer until the meat and vegetables are tender, 30 to 40 minutes longer.

6. Spoon the stew into four bowls and top each with parsley or thyme (if using).

Korean Barbecue Beef Lettuce Wraps

SERVES 4

Based on the traditional, semi-sweet Korean bulgogi *beef dish, this recipe has been modified to contain less sugar. Thin-sliced beef may be purchased at Asian markets, or purchase a larger cut from your local farmers' market, butcher, or natural grocery store and use a sharp knife to slice against the grain for paper-thin pieces. Partially freezing the beef beforehand makes slicing easier.*

- ⅓ CUP GLUTEN-FREE SOY SAUCE, SUCH AS TAMARI OR BRAGG LIQUID AMINOS
- 1 TABLESPOON SHERRY VINEGAR
- 1 TABLESPOON SESAME OIL
- 2 TABLESPOONS RAW HONEY, GRADE B PURE MAPLE SYRUP, OR AGAVE NECTAR
- 3 GARLIC CLOVES, MINCED
- 2 GREEN ONIONS, BOTH GREEN AND WHITE PARTS, FINELY SLICED
- 2 TABLESPOONS TOASTED SESAME SEEDS
- ¼ TEASPOON RED PEPPER FLAKES
- ¼ TEASPOON MINCED GINGER, OR MORE, IF DESIRED
- ¼ TEASPOON FRESHLY GROUND BLACK PEPPER
- 1½ POUNDS TOP SIRLOIN, FLAT IRON, FLANK, OR OTHER LEAN STEAK, THINLY SLICED
- ½ YELLOW ONION, THINLY SLICED
- 2 TABLESPOONS GRAPE-SEED, AVOCADO, OR COCONUT OIL
- 8 TO 10 LARGE BOSTON OR ROMAINE LETTUCE LEAVES
- 1 CUP GRATED CARROT
- 1 CUP GRATED CUCUMBER
- SRIRACHA SAUCE (OPTIONAL)

1. Combine the soy sauce, vinegar, sesame oil, honey, garlic, green onions, sesame seeds, red pepper flakes, ginger, and pepper in a large bowl.

continued ▶

Korean Barbecue Beef Lettuce Wraps *continued* ▶

2. Add the beef and onion slices and massage to coat the beef completely. Cover and refrigerate for 1 hour.

3. Drain the beef, discarding the marinade.

4. Heat the grape-seed oil in a large skillet over medium-high heat. Add half of the beef and onion in a single layer, and cook until the beef is slightly crispy, browned on the edges, and cooked through, turning once, about 2 minutes per side.

5. Set the cooked beef aside and repeat the cooking process with the remaining beef and onion.

6. Combine all the beef and onion and pour the residual pan juice over the beef.

7. Serve the beef immediately with lettuce leaves, carrots, cucumber, and Sriracha sauce (if using).

Argentinean Skirt Steak with Chimichurri

SERVES 4

Chimichurri is a classic South American condiment that pairs beautifully with steak. If you have any, this is a great recipe to use up any leftover steak—you won't regret it.

1½ TO 2 POUNDS SKIRT STEAK, CUT INTO 4 PIECES
½ TEASPOON SEA SALT
½ TEASPOON FRESHLY GROUND BLACK PEPPER
1 CUP CHIMICHURRI (PAGE 162)

1. Heat the grill to medium-high or heat a cast-iron grill pan over medium-high heat.

2. Season the steaks with salt and pepper.

3. Grill the steaks for 3 to 4 minutes per side for medium-rare doneness (about 135°F).

4. Serve the steaks with the Chimichurri.

Standing Rib Roast with Mustard-Horseradish Sauce

SERVES 6 TO 8

Standing rib roast sounds like a holiday-only, intimidating dish. In fact, it's easy to prepare and makes great leftovers for lunch and quick snacks. Serve it with green beans, sautéed greens, or a simple salad.

1 (3-RIB) STANDING BEEF RIB ROAST (ABOUT 6 POUNDS)
½ TEASPOON SEA SALT
1 TEASPOON FRESHLY GROUND BLACK PEPPER
⅓ CUP PREPARED HORSERADISH
2 TEASPOONS RED WINE VINEGAR
1 TABLESPOON DIJON MUSTARD

1. Preheat the oven to 400°F.

2. Place the roast, bones-side down, in a shallow roasting pan and season it with the salt and pepper.

3. Place the roast in the oven and immediately reduce the heat to 325°F. Bake the roast for 20 minutes per pound until the internal temperature of the meat reaches 120°F to 130°F for rare or 135°F to 145°F for medium doneness.

4. Remove the roast from the oven and let it stand on a carving board, tented with foil, for 20 minutes.

5. While the roast is cooking, combine the horseradish, vinegar, and mustard in a small bowl and whisk vigorously until creamy, or process the mixture in a blender. Refrigerate the sauce until serving time.

6. Remove the ribs from the roast and reserve them, if desired, to make a beef-based broth (see Chicken Broth recipe, page 158).

7. Carve the roast beef into thin slices and serve it with the horseradish sauce.

Tri-Colored Eggplant "Lasagna" with Sausage

SERVES 6

Since this is a pasta-free dish, baking the vegetables briefly first helps prevent the lasagna from becoming too watery. Freeze leftover lasagna squares for quick lunches and weeknight dinners.

2 (1-POUND) EGGPLANTS, ENDS TRIMMED, PEELED, AND CUT LENGTHWISE INTO ¼-INCH-THICK SLICES
4 TABLESPOONS EXTRA-VIRGIN OLIVE OIL
1 TEASPOON SEA SALT
2 LARGE RED, GREEN, AND/OR YELLOW BELL PEPPERS, QUARTERED LENGTHWISE
1 POUND HOT OR MILD ITALIAN SAUSAGE, CASINGS REMOVED
3 CUPS TOMATO SAUCE (PAGE 157)
½ TEASPOON RED CHILI FLAKES (OPTIONAL)
3 CUPS BABY SPINACH LEAVES
1 CUP ITALIAN PINE NUTS
½ CUP CHOPPED FRESH BASIL, THINLY SLICED, FOR GARNISH

1. Preheat the oven to 400°F.

2. Place the eggplant slices on a large rimmed baking sheet in a single layer. Brush 2 tablespoons of the olive oil over the eggplant; then sprinkle them with ½ teaspoon of the salt.

3. Turn the slices over and brush them with the remaining 2 tablespoons of oil. Sprinkle them with the remaining ½ teaspoon of salt.

4. Arrange the pepper quarters around the eggplant (they do not need to be dressed with the oil). Bake until the vegetables begin to soften and release their juices, 5 to 10 minutes.

5. Reduce the oven temperature to 375°F.

continued ▶

Tri-Colored Eggplant "Lasagna" with Sausage *continued* ▶

6. Meanwhile, crumble the sausage into a skillet. Cook over medium heat until browned, stirring frequently, about 5 minutes.

7. Add the Tomato Sauce and red chili flakes (if using), and simmer for 5 minutes.

8. Cover the bottom of a 13-by-9-inch glass baking dish with a layer of sausage sauce.

9. Layer half of the eggplant and pepper quarters over the sauce. Top the eggplant with 1 cup of the spinach and 1 cup of the sausage sauce, spread evenly over the first layer.

10. Repeat the layers with the remaining eggplant, peppers, spinach, and sauce. Spoon any remaining sauce over the top; then sprinkle the lasagna with pine nuts.

11. Bake the dish uncovered until bubbly, 25 to 35 minutes.

12. Remove the lasagna from the oven, cut it into squares, and serve with basil garnish.

Italian Sausage–Stuffed Peppers

SERVES 4

Just like the classic dish you'll find in many Italian restaurants, this Paleo-friendly version satisfies with the same great taste but double the vegetables.

4 RED, YELLOW, AND/OR GREEN BELL PEPPERS
1 POUND HOT OR MILD ITALIAN SAUSAGE, CASINGS REMOVED
1 YELLOW ONION, CHOPPED
2 CUPS TOMATO SAUCE (PAGE 157)
½ CUP CHOPPED FRESH BASIL, PLUS MORE FOR GARNISH, IF DESIRED
1 TEASPOON DRIED OREGANO
6 CUPS PACKED BABY SPINACH LEAVES

1. Preheat the oven to 375°F.

2. Cut off the tops of the bell peppers about ¾ of an inch from the top, and slice off a small portion of the bottom to allow the bell peppers to stand upright. Chop the bell pepper tops, discarding the stems. Clean out and discard the seeds and membrane from the bell peppers and set them aside.

3. Crumble the sausage into a large skillet and cook it for 3 minutes.

4. Add the onion and chopped bell pepper and cook for 5 to 6 minutes or until the meat is no longer pink.

5. Add the Tomato Sauce, basil, and oregano. Bring the mixture to a simmer and cook for 4 minutes.

6. Use tongs to add the spinach in batches, turning it just until each batch is wilted.

7. Stand the bell peppers up in an 8-inch glass baking dish or casserole dish. Spoon the filling into the bell peppers, and bake them for 30 minutes or until the bell peppers are tender and the filling is heated through.

8. Serve topped with additional basil (if using).

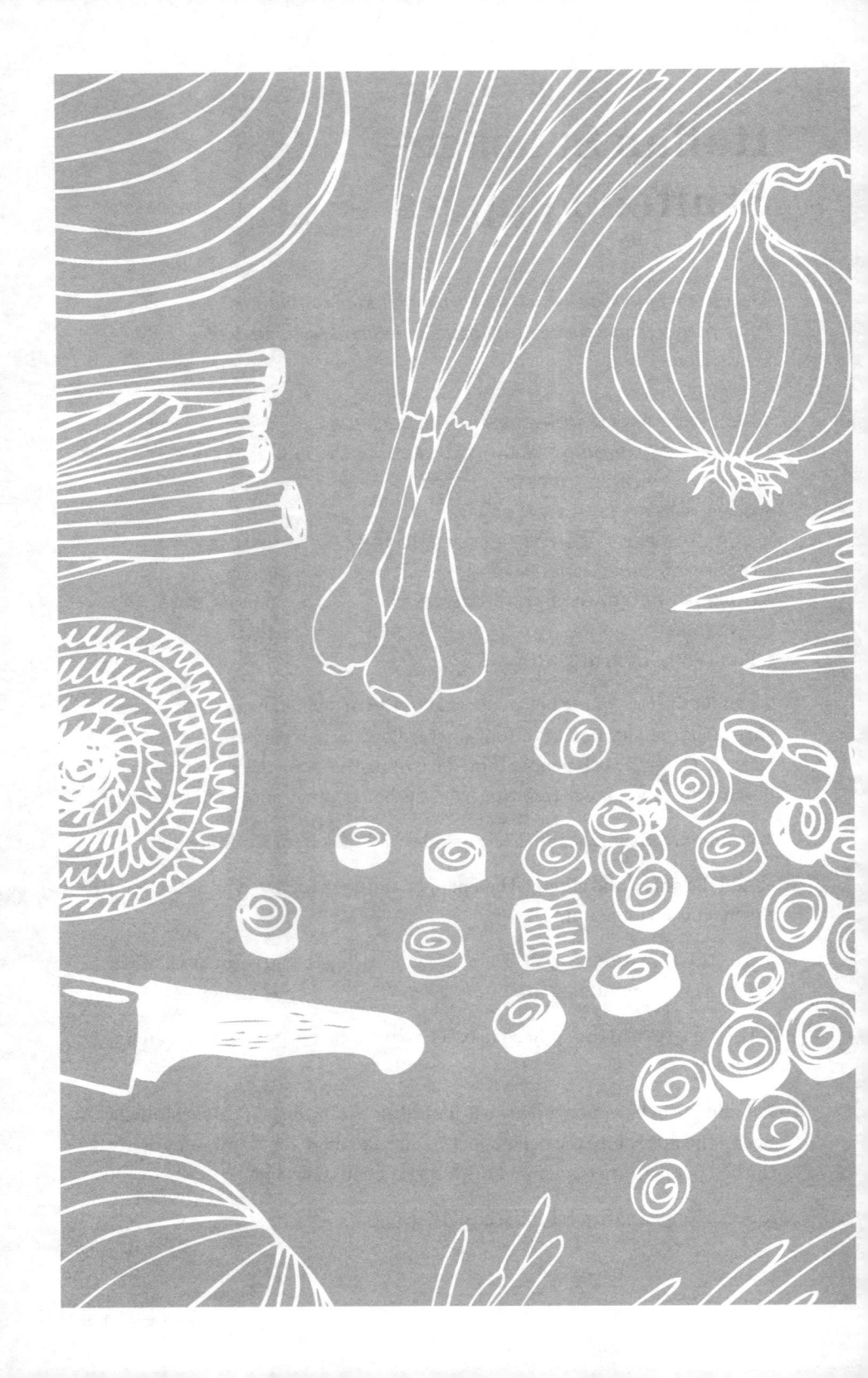

CHAPTER NINE

Dessert

CHIA SEED PUDDING

PUMPKIN CUSTARD

CHOCOLATE COCONUT TRUFFLES

QUICK AND EASY MICROWAVE BROWNIE

COCONUT DATE "BLONDIES"

ALMOND BUTTER BITES

CHOCOLATE CHIP COOKIES

BLUEBERRY MACADAMIA SQUARES

CHOCOLATE-CHERRY BARK

ALMOND BUTTER CUPS

PALEO "CHEESECAKE"

COCONUT WHIPPED CREAM

CHOCOLATE-STRAWBERRY "MILK" SHAKE

COCONUT VANILLA ICE CREAM

HORCHATA ICE POPS

VERY BERRY GRANITA

Chia Seed Pudding

SERVES 4

Missing the creamy texture of yogurt? Chia seed "pudding" stands in as a quick fix enriched with protein and healthful fat but without the dairy. The seeds start off small but plump up as they absorb the almond or coconut milk, creating a tapioca-like consistency. Aside from dessert, chia seed pudding makes for a great snack or satisfying breakfast when combined with extra berries, protein, and/or nuts.

1¾ CUPS UNSWEETENED ALMOND OR COCONUT MILK
2 TABLESPOONS RAW HONEY, GRADE B MAPLE SYRUP,
    OR AGAVE NECTAR
¼ CUP CHIA SEEDS
1 TEASPOON PURE VANILLA EXTRACT OR 1 WHOLE VANILLA BEAN
1 TABLESPOON RAW CACAO POWDER (OPTIONAL)

1. In a large glass jar or bowl, whisk together the milk, honey, seeds, and extract. If using a vanilla bean, score the length of the pod with the tip of a knife to expose the beans and drop the beans into the mixture.

2. Add cacao (if using). Whisk to combine.

3. Cover and refrigerate the pudding for at least 4 hours or overnight. Stir after the first 30 minutes to redistribute the seeds and again after 3 hours or the next morning if they have settled on the bottom and the pudding has not thickened fully.

4. Discard the vanilla beans before serving.

5. Serve the pudding chilled, and store leftovers in the refrigerator for up to 3 days.

Pumpkin Custard

SERVES 4

As delicious as the pie, this crustless custard has all the flavors you crave without the guilt. The mixture may also work as a base for ice cream. Leftover pumpkin may be frozen for later use.

2 CUPS WATER
1¼ CUPS COCONUT MILK
4 EGGS
½ CUP GRADE B MAPLE SYRUP OR AGAVE NECTAR
¾ CUP CANNED PUMPKIN PURÉE (NOT PUMPKIN PIE FILLING)
1 TEASPOON GROUND CINNAMON
½ TEASPOON GROUND NUTMEG
½ TEASPOON PURE VANILLA EXTRACT
⅛ TEASPOON SEA SALT

1. Preheat the oven to 325°F.

2. In a saucepan, bring the water to a boil.

3. Heat the milk in a small saucepot over medium heat until it is simmering but not boiling.

4. In a separate bowl, whisk together the eggs and syrup.

5. Very slowly pour the warm milk into the egg mixture, whisking constantly.

6. Add the pumpkin and remaining ingredients and whisk well.

7. Pour the mixture into 4 ramekins or small, disposable foil tins. Set the ramekins into a 9-by-13-inch baking dish and pour the boiling water around the ramekins until it reaches halfway up the sides of the ramekins.

8. Bake the custard for 30 minutes or until a toothpick inserted in the middle comes out clean.

9. Serve the custard warm or chilled.

Chocolate Coconut Truffles

MAKES 12 TRUFFLES

Simple to make and easy to keep, these truffles make a delicious and quick treat.

2 CUPS PITTED MEDJOOL DATES
6 TABLESPOONS UNSWEETENED COCONUT FLAKES, PLUS MORE FOR DUSTING
3 TABLESPOONS COCONUT OIL
2 TABLESPOONS RAW HONEY
2 TABLESPOONS UNSWEETENED COCOA OR RAW CACAO POWDER

1. Combine all of the ingredients in a food processor and blend until sticky.

2. Roll the mixture into balls and place them on a parchment-lined plate.

3. Cover the balls with additional coconut flakes, if desired.

4. Chill until the truffles are firm. The truffles will last up to 3 months in the freezer.

Quick and Easy Microwave Brownie

SERVES 1

No need to get out the baking equipment for this easy brownie-like dessert. This recipe is perfect for days when you need a comforting end-of-meal treat.

2 TABLESPOONS ALMOND BUTTER
2 TABLESPOONS WATER
¼ TEASPOON PURE VANILLA EXTRACT
2 TABLESPOONS UNSWEETENED COCOA OR RAW CACAO POWDER
1½ TABLESPOONS RAW HONEY, GRADE B MAPLE SYRUP, OR AGAVE NECTAR
4 TABLESPOONS ALMOND MEAL

1. In a 12-ounce mug, whisk together the almond butter, water, and vanilla.

2. Add the cocoa powder, honey, and almond meal. Whisk until fully combined.

3. Microwave the mug on high for 60 to 90 seconds for a slightly molten center.

4. Serve the brownie with a spoon and Coconut Whipped Cream (page 149), if desired.

Coconut Date "Blondies"

MAKES ABOUT 16 BARS

Sometimes you want a blondie over a brownie. This bakeless Paleo version uses dates as a natural sweetener, and plenty of coconut for a rich, guiltless treat.

1½ CUPS UNSALTED RAW CASHEWS
1½ CUPS PITTED MEDJOOL DATES
½ CUP ALMOND BUTTER
½ CUP ALMOND MEAL
½ CUP UNSWEETENED COCONUT FLAKES, PLUS MORE FOR TOPPING
1½ TABLESPOONS COCONUT OIL, MELTED
¼ TEASPOON PURE VANILLA EXTRACT

1. Add the cashews, dates, and almond butter to a food processor or blender and process until mixed.

2. Add the almond meal, coconut flakes, oil, and vanilla extract. Process until a thick dough forms.

3. Press the dough into the bottom of an 8-by-8-inch square baking pan and top with extra coconut flakes.

4. Refrigerate the blondies for 6 hours or overnight. Cut it into square bars and serve. Leftovers can be stored in the refrigerator for up to 3 days or in the freezer for about 2 months.

Almond Butter Bites

MAKES 12 BALLS

These no-bake treats can easily stand in as a quick, on-the-go breakfast or light snack. Remember to store ground flaxseed in the refrigerator once it's opened.

1 CUP ALMOND MEAL
½ CUP GROUND FLAXSEED
½ CUP UNSALTED RAW OR ROASTED ALMOND BUTTER
2 TABLESPOONS RAW HONEY, GRADE B PURE MAPLE SYRUP, OR AGAVE NECTAR
½ TEASPOON GROUND CINNAMON
¼ CUP RAW CACAO POWDER (OPTIONAL)

1. Combine all of the ingredients except the cacao powder in a bowl. Stir until it is well combined.

2. Roll the dough into balls and arrange them on a parchment-lined sheet, tray, or plate. Refrigerate the bites until they are firm, about 1 hour.

3. Roll the balls in cacao powder (if using), shaking to remove any excess powder.

4. Store the bites in the freezer for up to 3 months.

Chocolate Chip Cookies

MAKES 12 COOKIES

Every diet should make room for chocolate chip cookies. These Paleo-friendly cookies are every bit as good as the classic cookies you love, but without the wheat and added sugar.

1¼ CUPS ALMOND FLOUR
⅛ TEASPOON SALT
⅛ TEASPOON BAKING SODA
5 TABLESPOONS COCONUT OIL, MELTED
½ TABLESPOON PURE VANILLA EXTRACT
½ CUP RAW HONEY, GRADE B PURE MAPLE SYRUP, OR AGAVE NECTAR
1 CUP CHOPPED UNSWEETENED CHOCOLATE OR CHOPPED CHOCOLATE-CHERRY BARK (PAGE 146)

1. Combine the almond flour, salt, and baking soda in a large bowl.

2. In a separate bowl, stir together the oil, vanilla, and honey.

3. Add the wet ingredients to the dry ingredients.

4. Fold in the chocolate pieces.

5. Shape the dough into 1-inch balls and place them 2 inches apart on a baking sheet lined with foil or greased with coconut oil.

6. Bake the cookies for 7 to 10 minutes or until browned. Transfer the cookies to a cooling rack.

7. Serve the cookies warm or at room temperature. Store leftover cookies in the freezer.

Blueberry Macadamia Squares

MAKES 16 SQUARES

Fruity and delicious, this easy-to-make dessert may be stored in the freezer for a quick, sweet bite. The blueberry topping may also be used like a Paleo-friendly jam to pair with almond butter for snacks and at breakfast.

2 CUPS UNSALTED LIGHTLY TOASTED MACADAMIA NUTS
½ CUP PITTED MEDJOOL DATES
¼ CUP UNSWEETENED COCONUT FLAKES
1 POUND FROZEN BLUEBERRIES
2 TABLESPOONS RAW HONEY, GRADE B PURE MAPLE SYRUP, OR AGAVE NECTAR
DASH OF GROUND CINNAMON (OPTIONAL)

1. Place the nuts, dates, and coconut flakes in a food processor or blender, and process until a sticky crumb consistency forms.

2. Transfer the mixture to a 9-by-9-inch baking pan. Press it evenly into the bottom to form a crust.

3. Heat a small saucepan over medium heat. Add the blueberries and cook until the berries begin to break down and release juices, about 5 minutes. Continue to cook until the berries thicken like a jam, being careful not to scorch or burn the bottom, 3 to 5 minutes.

4. Stir in the honey and cinnamon (if using). Cook for 30 seconds more until the ingredients are well combined.

5. Remove the mixture from the heat and allow it to cool for 10 minutes.

6. Pour the blueberry mixture on top of the crust, spreading it evenly to distribute it throughout the pan. Refrigerate until it is firm, about 1 hour.

7. Cut the pie into 2-by-2-inch squares and enjoy. Store leftover squares in the freezer for up to 3 months.

Chocolate-Cherry Bark

MAKES ABOUT 32 SQUARES

The add-in options for this chocolate bark are endless. Try other dried unsweetened fruits, different nuts, almond butter, and even goji berries and cacao nibs. Look for raw cacao paste in "bark" form at natural grocery and health food stores, but if it's not available, unsweetened chocolate works just fine.

1 POUND UNSWEETENED CHOCOLATE OR RAW CACAO PASTE, CHOPPED
¼ CUP RAW HONEY, GRADE B PURE MAPLE SYRUP, OR AGAVE NECTAR
3 TABLESPOONS DRIED UNSWEETENED CHERRIES
2 TABLESPOONS UNSALTED NUTS (OPTIONAL)
2 TO 3 TABLESPOONS UNSWEETENED COCONUT FLAKES (OPTIONAL)

1. Line a 9-by-9-inch baking pan or other small sheet tray with heavy-duty aluminum foil. Crimp the edges of the foil around the pan to create a square with ½-inch-high sides.

2. Prepare a double boiler by setting a large stainless steel bowl over a saucepot with boiling water. Add half of the chocolate to the bowl, stirring frequently with a wooden spoon. Once the chocolate is melted, add the remaining chocolate a little at a time.

3. Once all the chocolate is completely melted, add the honey, cherries, and nuts (if using). Mix well.

4. Pour the mixture evenly into the foil and spread it with a rubber spatula until smooth. Top the mixture with coconut flakes (if using).

5. Transfer the baking pan to the refrigerator and allow the bark to cool for 1 hour.

6. Cut the chocolate into approximately 1-by-1-inch squares for ½-ounce pieces. Store the bark in the freezer in a heavy-duty resealable plastic bag or small tin for up to 3 months.

Almond Butter Cups

MAKES ABOUT 8 CUPS

Just like those peanut butter cups you crave, these Paleo treats will give you that chocolate–nut butter fix with a healthier spin. Store the cups in the freezer, cutting them in half to reduce the portion size, if desired.

8 OUNCES UNSWEETENED DARK CHOCOLATE, CHOPPED
4 TABLESPOONS RAW HONEY, GRADE B PURE MAPLE SYRUP, OR AGAVE NECTAR
½ CUP ALMOND BUTTER
½ TEASPOON PURE VANILLA EXTRACT
⅛ TEASPOON SEA SALT

1. Line an 8-cup muffin pan with paper liners.

2. Prepare a double boiler by setting a large, stainless steel bowl over a saucepot with boiling water. Add half of the chocolate to the bowl, stirring frequently with a wooden spoon. Once the chocolate is melted, add the remaining chocolate a little at a time.

3. Once all the chocolate is completely melted, add 2 tablespoons of the honey.

4. In a small bowl, mix together the remaining 2 tablespoons of honey, almond butter, vanilla, and salt. If the mixture is too thick to easily combine, microwave it for 10 seconds.

5. Using a brush or spoon, spread about 1 tablespoon of chocolate in the bottom of each liner, brushing the chocolate upward about 1 inch to partially cover the sides.

6. Spoon about 1 tablespoon of the almond butter mixture into each cup. Make sure all cups have an even amount of the mixture.

7. Divide the remaining chocolate evenly among the cups, spreading it lightly to cover the almond butter mixture.

8. Transfer the muffin pan to the freezer for at least 1 hour to set.

9. Remove the cups from the pan and peel back the liners to enjoy.

Paleo "Cheesecake"

SERVES 8 TO 12

This nuttier version of the dairy original tastes just as great, if not better. The bakeless crust shaves hours off the prep time and may be used as a great neutral base for other Paleo-friendly toppings, tarts, and cakes.

FOR THE CRUST:
1¼ CUPS WALNUTS
1¼ CUPS UNSALTED TOASTED CASHEWS
1½ CUPS PITTED MEDJOOL DATES
1 TEASPOON GROUND CINNAMON

FOR THE CHEESECAKE FILLING:
1½ CUPS RAW UNSALTED CASHEWS, SOAKED FOR 4 HOURS AND DRIED
6 TABLESPOONS COCONUT OIL, MELTED
2 TABLESPOONS FRESH LEMON JUICE
¼ CUP RAW HONEY, GRADE B PURE MAPLE SYRUP, OR AGAVE NECTAR
1 TEASPOON PURE VANILLA EXTRACT
6 TABLESPOONS FILTERED WATER
MIXED FRESH BERRIES (OPTIONAL)

To make the crust:

1. Place all the ingredients in a food processor or blender and process until a sticky crumb consistency forms.

2. Transfer mixture to an 8-inch pie pan. Press it evenly into the bottom to form a crust.

To make the cheesecake filling:

1. Add the cashews, coconut oil, lemon juice, honey, vanilla extract, and water to the food processor or blender. Process until very smooth.

2. Pour the mixture onto the crust and freeze the cheesecake for 1 to 2 hours.

3. When it is firm, slice the frozen cheesecake into 8 or 12 wedges. Serve it thawed with berries (if using). Store leftover slices in the freezer for up to 3 months.

Coconut Whipped Cream

MAKES ABOUT 1¼ TO 1½ CUPS

Add this extra bit of sweetness to the Chocolate-Strawberry "Milk" Shake (page 150), an ice cream sundae, or your favorite pie or cobbler.

1 (14-OUNCE) CAN FULL-FAT COCONUT MILK, CHILLED

1. Turn the can upside down and remove the lid. Pour the milky white liquid into a bowl, stopping at the thickened coconut mixture at the bottom of the can. Discard white liquid.

2. Scoop the thickened coconut into a separate bowl and whip it with a hand mixer. Alternately, transfer the thickened coconut cream to a stand mixer and whip until frothy. Cover and chill the whipped cream until use.

Chocolate-Strawberry "Milk" Shake

SERVES 2

Tasty for dessert or breakfast, this creamy shake easily stands in for any dairy version.

2 CUPS FROZEN STRAWBERRIES
1 CUP UNSWEETENED ALMOND OR COCONUT MILK, CHILLED
2 TABLESPOONS RAW CACAO POWDER
1 TABLESPOON RAW HONEY, GRADE B PURE MAPLE SYRUP, OR AGAVE NECTAR

1. Combine all of the ingredients in a blender and blend on high until it is smooth and combined.

2. Pour the shake into two glasses and serve immediately.

Coconut Vanilla Ice Cream

SERVES 4

Start with this base and build from there. Great on its own, this ice cream also works well with unsweetened coconut flakes, nuts, and dried fruit as toppings. Or pair it with other Paleo desserts in this chapter, like Almond Butter Cups (page 147), Chocolate-Cherry Bark (page 166), and Coconut Whipped Cream (page 149).

1 (13.5-OUNCE) CAN COCONUT MILK
4 EGG YOLKS
2 TABLESPOONS RAW HONEY, GRADE B PURE MAPLE SYRUP, OR AGAVE NECTAR
1 TEASPOON PURE VANILLA EXTRACT

1. Prepare a double boiler by setting a large, stainless steel bowl over a saucepot with boiling water. Add the coconut milk and bring it to a simmer, but be careful not to boil the milk.

2. Meanwhile, whisk together the egg yolks, honey, and vanilla.

3. Add one-third of the hot milk into the egg mixture, whisking constantly.

4. Repeat until all the milk is combined with the egg mixture; then transfer the mixture back to the double boiler.

5. Whisking constantly, continue to cook the mixture over medium heat until the ice cream base has thickened enough to coat the back of a spoon. Pour the mixture into a bowl and cool it completely in the refrigerator.

6. Pour the mixture into an ice cream maker, and prepare the ice cream according to the manufacturer's directions.

7. Freeze the ice cream for an additional 2 hours to serve hardened, if desired.

Horchata Ice Pops

SERVES 2 TO 4

Inspired by the traditional cinnamon-spiked Mexican beverage, this Paleo version skips all the sugar. If you don't have ice-pop molds, you can make your own: Pour the horchata into small disposable cups covered with a sheet of aluminum foil; then pierce the foil with wooden sticks and insert them into the cups so they stand upright.

3 CUPS UNSWEETENED ALMOND MILK
¼ CUP RAW HONEY, GRADE B PURE MAPLE SYRUP, OR AGAVE NECTAR
1 TABLESPOON GROUND CINNAMON
1½ TEASPOONS PURE VANILLA EXTRACT OR SEEDS FROM 1 VANILLA BEAN POD
¼ TEASPOON GROUND NUTMEG

1. Place all the ingredients in a blender and process for 30 seconds on high.

2. Pour the horchata into ice-pop molds and freeze until firm, 2 to 3 hours.

3. To serve, place the ice-pop tray or mold under warm running water for a few seconds to loosen the horchata, and then remove the pops.

Very Berry Granita

SERVES 4 TO 8

Snow cone–like granitas are extra easy to make because they only require freezing with the occasional stirring. Bright and refreshing, this Paleo-friendly version skips refined sugar for the natural sweetness of fruit with a touch of honey.

1¼ CUPS FILTERED WATER
½ CUP RAW HONEY, GRADE B PURE MAPLE SYRUP, OR AGAVE NECTAR
½ TEASPOON LEMON ZEST
4 CUPS FRESH OR FROZEN MIXED BERRIES (BLUEBERRIES, RASPBERRIES, AND/OR STRAWBERRIES)
1 TEASPOON FRESH LEMON JUICE
CHOPPED FRESH MINT LEAVES (OPTIONAL)

1. Bring the water, honey, and lemon zest to a boil in a medium saucepot. Remove the saucepot from the heat and let it stand for 5 minutes.

2. Pour the mixture into a bowl and refrigerate it until it's cool, about 45 minutes.

3. Puree berries and lemon juice in a food processor or blender until smooth.

4. Add the berry mixture to the sweetened water mixture and mix well.

5. Pour the granita base into a 9-by-13-inch metal baking pan.

6. Freeze the granita until ice crystals form around edges of pan, about 30 minutes. Using a spoon, scrape up the ice crystals and stir them back into the mixture.

7. Freeze the granita for another 1 to 1½ hours, stirring every 30 minutes, until the entire mixture is frozen.

8. Scoop out ½ to 1 cup portions and serve them with mint leaves (if using).

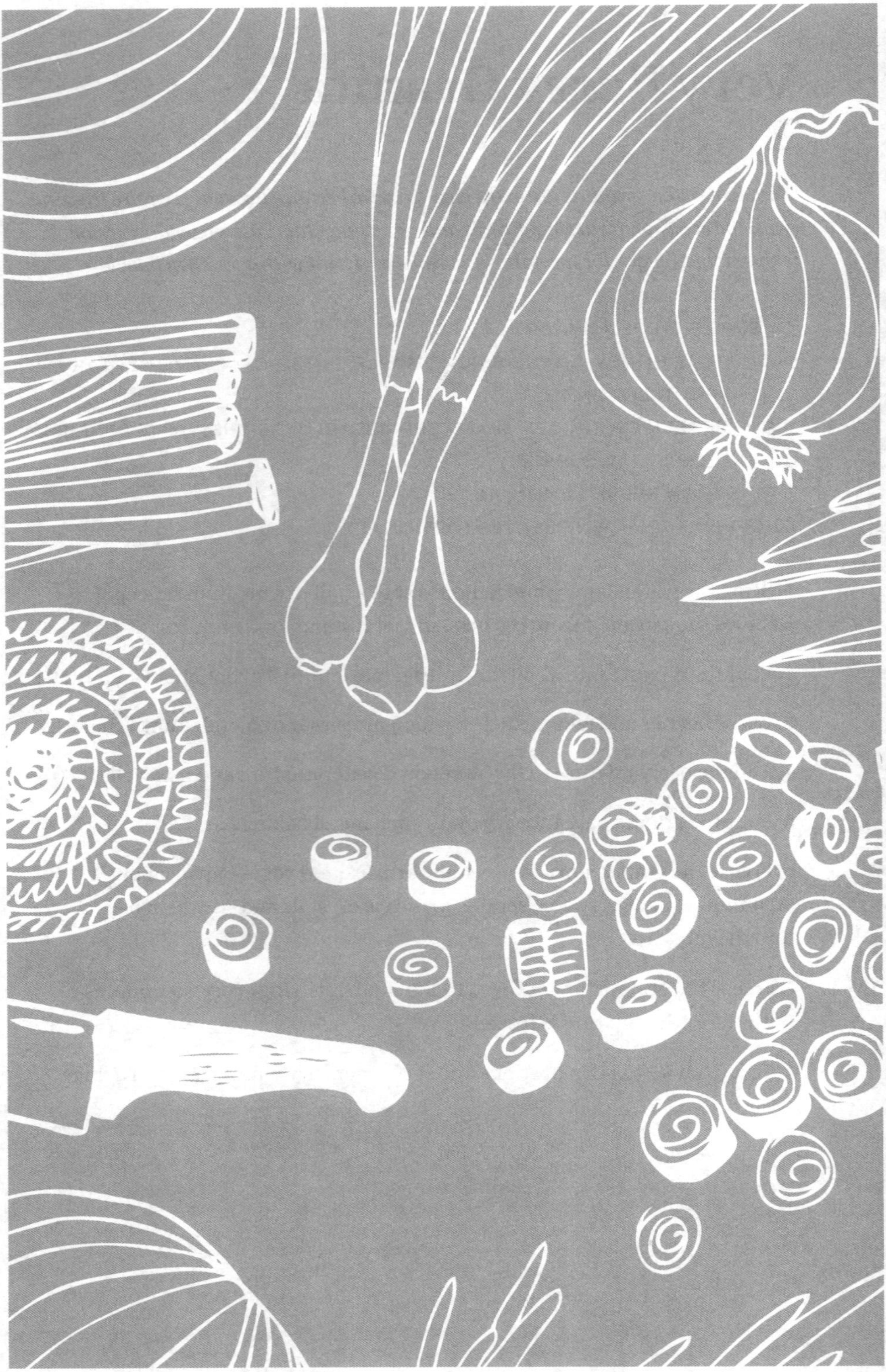

CHAPTER TEN

Pantry Recipes

The Paleo lifestyle is all about paying close attention to the food you buy as well as making a lot of your own to control sodium and sugar and avoid additives and preservatives.

This chapter contains easy recipes for staples you can make yourself to keep on hand for months or, in some cases, longer in the freezer. Gather glass jars and freezer-safe containers and bags to store your homemade goodies. Pantry recipes include:

- NUT BUTTER
- TOMATO SAUCE
- CHICKEN BROTH
- CREAMY SALAD DRESSING
- PESTO
- CHIMICHURRI
- MAYONNAISE
- HARD-BOILED EGGS
- GUACAMOLE
- ROASTED TOMATO SALSA

Nut Butter

MAKES ABOUT 1 CUP

While some health food stores carry unsalted nut butters, you can easily make your own using a good-quality food processor or blender. It is possible to make nut butter without any added oil, but running the processor for long periods of time may risk burning out the motor.

2 TO 4 CUPS UNSALTED ROASTED ALMONDS, CASHEWS, AND/OR HAZELNUTS

1 TO 2 TABLESPOONS WALNUT OIL

1. Add the nuts to the blender and blend them on high until they are very fine and the nuts begin to release their oils, 3 to 5 minutes. Pay attention to the processor to make sure it is not overheating.

2. Add the walnut oil 1 tablespoon at a time, as needed, and continue to blend the nuts until the mixture becomes creamy. Store it in an airtight jar in the refrigerator for up to 1 month.

Tomato Sauce

MAKES 3 TO 4 CUPS

Many prepared tomato sauces have excessive amounts of sodium as well as hidden sugars and other additives. Make your own by using fresh, ripened tomatoes when in season, or look for tomatoes packaged in boxes rather than cans, if possible, to avoid potential BPA contamination.

2 TABLESPOONS EXTRA-VIRGIN OLIVE OIL
1 YELLOW ONION, FINELY CHOPPED
4 GARLIC CLOVES, MINCED
1 (26-OUNCE) BOX WHOLE OR CRUSHED NO-SALT-ADDED TOMATOES OR 10 VINE-RIPENED, HEIRLOOM, SAN MARZANO, OR OTHER RED-COLORED FRESH TOMATOES, BOILED, PEELED, AND CHOPPED
1 TABLESPOON DRIED OREGANO
1 TABLESPOON FRESH OR DRIED THYME
½ TEASPOON FRESHLY GROUND BLACK PEPPER

1. Add the oil to a large skillet over medium-high heat, and cook the onion until soft and translucent, about 2 minutes.

2. Add the garlic and cook until fragrant, 1 minute.

3. Add the tomatoes, herbs, and pepper. Bring to a simmer and cook until the sauce thickens, about 10 minutes or longer.

4. Allow the sauce to cool for 10 minutes; then chill it in the refrigerator. For long-term storage, freeze the sauce in individually portioned, resealable plastic bags or freezer-safe glass containers for up to 3 months.

Chicken Broth

MAKES ABOUT 1 QUART

This basic recipe is a great staple to have on hand when you want to avoid the salt-laden stocks from the grocery store, or if low-sodium varieties are not available. It also makes great use of your leftover chicken bones so they don't go to waste. Make sure your hood fan is working properly and on high speed to avoid stinking up your kitchen. For a vegetarian version, omit the chicken and double the amounts of onion, carrots, and celery.

3 TABLESPOONS EXTRA-VIRGIN OLIVE OIL
CHICKEN BONES AND CARCASS FROM ONE WHOLE CHICKEN
1 YELLOW ONION, DICED
3 CARROTS, PEELED AND DICED
3 CELERY STALKS, DICED
2 GARLIC CLOVES, CHOPPED
½ TEASPOON FRESHLY GROUND BLACK PEPPER
2 BAY LEAVES
5 SPRIGS THYME
WATER TO COVER (ABOUT 4 TO 6 QUARTS)

1. Heat 1 tablespoon of the oil in a large stockpot over medium-high heat, and add the chicken bones and scraps. Cook until the scraps are browned, turning occasionally, about 5 minutes. Remove the chicken pieces and set them aside.

2. Add remaining 2 tablespoons of oil and cook the onion until soft and translucent, about 2 minutes.

3. Add the carrots and celery, cooking until softened, 5 to 7 minutes. In the last minute of cooking, add the garlic and cook until fragrant.

4. Return the chicken bones and scraps to the pot, and add the pepper and herbs. Pour in enough water to cover everything.

5. Bring the stock to a boil. Reduce the heat and maintain a slow-rolling simmer for at least 1 hour, occasionally skimming off the fat with a spoon as it collects at the top.

6. Allow the stock to cool for 15 minutes, and then refrigerate it.

7. Skim and discard additional fat from the top of the broth before use. Freeze individual portions of the broth in resealable plastic bags or freezer-safe glass containers, if desired, for up to 4 months.

Creamy Salad Dressing

MAKES 1 CUP

Most salad dressings have a ratio of three parts oil to one part vinegar or other acid, such as lemon juice. Mustard acts as an emulsifier, blending both into a creamier consistency and extending the storage life of the dressing.

¾ CUP EXTRA-VIRGIN OLIVE, WALNUT, OR AVOCADO OIL
¼ CUP APPLE CIDER, RED WINE, OR BALSAMIC VINEGAR OR LEMON JUICE
½ TABLESPOON DIJON MUSTARD
⅛ TEASPOON SEA SALT
¼ TEASPOON FRESHLY GROUND BLACK PEPPER
1 TEASPOON CHOPPED FRESH THYME LEAVES (OPTIONAL)

1. Add all the ingredients to a resealable glass jar and shake vigorously until creamy.

2. Store the dressing in the refrigerator for up to 2 weeks. Shake the dressing again before each use to ensure it is well combined.

Pesto

MAKES 1 CUP

Though pesto traditional means a blend of basil, pine nuts, and Parmesan cheese, you may easily skip the cheese and try different herbs, nuts, and oils for different variations.

2 CUPS PACKED FRESH BASIL LEAVES OR 1 BUNCH PARSLEY, STEMMED
¼ CUP PINE NUTS OR WALNUTS
1 GARLIC CLOVE
⅔ CUP EXTRA-VIRGIN OLIVE, WALNUT, OR ALMOND OIL
PINCH OF SEA SALT
PINCH OF FRESHLY GROUND BLACK PEPPER

1. Put all of the ingredients into a blender or food processor and process until creamy.

2. Store the pesto in the refrigerator for up to 1 week. If the pesto hardens, let it sit at room temperature for 10 to 15 minutes and shake before use.

Chimichurri

MAKES ABOUT 1 CUP

This Argentinean sauce goes great with steak, fish, and other proteins. For an easier or creamier preparation, skip chopping the herbs and pulse the sauce in a blender two to three times. Though traditionally made with parsley, cilantro works well as a substitute.

1 CUP PACKED FRESH FLAT-LEAF PARSLEY OR CILANTRO, STEMMED AND FINELY CHOPPED

3 TO 4 GARLIC CLOVES, FINELY CHOPPED

2 TABLESPOONS CHOPPED FRESH OREGANO LEAVES OR 2 TEASPOONS DRIED OREGANO

½ CUP EXTRA-VIRGIN OLIVE, WALNUT, OR AVOCADO OIL

2 TABLESPOONS RED WINE VINEGAR

¼ TEASPOON SEA SALT

¼ TEASPOON FRESHLY GROUND BLACK PEPPER

¼ TEASPOON RED PEPPER FLAKES

1. Whisk together all the ingredients or combine them in a jar and shake vigorously.

2. Serve the sauce immediately or refrigerate it for up to 1 week. If it hardens, let it sit at room temperature for 10 to 15 minutes and shake before use.

Mayonnaise

MAKES ABOUT 1 CUP

Many commercial mayonnaise brands contain added sugars, salt, and preservatives. Make your own fresher version, but take care when using raw eggs. Consider using a pasteurized egg for this recipe, or boil the egg in 140°F water for three minutes, using a thermometer to make sure the water temperature is consistent. Discard the egg white.

1 PASTEURIZED EGG YOLK
JUICE OF ½ LEMON
½ TEASPOON DIJON MUSTARD
PINCH OF SEA SALT
¾ CUP EXTRA-VIRGIN OLIVE, WALNUT, OR AVOCADO OIL

1. Add all the ingredients except the oil to a food processor or blender. Pulse two times to lightly mix.

2. Add the oil and process until smooth and creamy.

3. Store the mayonnaise in the refrigerator for up to 2 days.

Hard-Boiled Eggs

MAKES 6 EGGS

Grocery stores carry bags of hard-boiled eggs, but making your own ensures you'll always have a quick snack or breakfast ready. When you run out of fresh eggs, save your egg carton to store unpeeled hard-boiled eggs.

6 EGGS

1. Add the eggs to a saucepan and cover them with cold water. Bring the water to a boil. Turn off the heat, cover, and let sit for 12 minutes.

2. Remove the eggs with a slotted spoon and transfer them to a bowl filled with ice water. When cooled, peel the eggs, running them under cold water, if necessary, to make the peeling easier.

3. Store the eggs in the refrigerator for up to 5 days.

Guacamole

MAKES ABOUT 2 CUPS

A Paleo staple, this healthful-fat condiment works great as a topper for eggs, meat, and seafood or as a dip for crunchy raw vegetables—no chips necessary.

3 AVOCADOS, PEELED, SEEDED, AND DICED
JUICE FROM ½ LIME
1 JALAPEÑO OR SERRANO PEPPER, SEEDED AND MINCED
2 TO 3 TABLESPOONS MINCED RED ONION
½ BUNCH (ABOUT ¼ CUP) CILANTRO, STEMS REMOVED AND FINELY CHOPPED
PINCH OF SEA SALT

1. In a large bowl, mash the avocado and lime juice with a spoon or pestle until the avocado is just slightly chunky.

2. Fold in the jalapeño pepper, onion, and cilantro. Season with the salt, if needed.

3. Chill the guacamole, covered, for 20 minutes or serve it immediately with cucumber slices and/or red and yellow bell pepper strips.

4. For variations, add roasted garlic, toasted pumpkin seeds, a touch of salsa, and/or broiled, peeled, and chopped tomatoes and chiles.

Roasted Tomato Salsa

MAKES ABOUT 1½ CUPS

Store-bought salsas often contain hidden additives and sugar. Making your own is easy and a great way to make use of extra tomatoes and peppers when they're in season. Store salsa in the refrigerator for two weeks or freeze it in individual portions for long-term storage up to six months.

1 POUND TOMATOES
1 TO 2 JALAPEÑO OR SERRANO PEPPERS
2 GARLIC CLOVES, UNPEELED
½ RED ONION
1 TABLESPOON WATER (OPTIONAL)
PINCH OF SEA SALT (OPTIONAL)

1. Preheat the broiler to high heat.

2. Place the vegetables on an aluminum foil–lined baking sheet and broil them 4 to 5 inches from heat source until blackened, about 10 minutes, turning once or twice.

3. Remove the vegetables from the oven, cover them with foil, and let them stand for 10 minutes.

4. Remove and discard the tomato and pepper skins, transferring the flesh and juices from the foil to a food processor or blender.

5. Squeeze the garlic from their shells into the food processor.

6. Remove and discard the outer layer of the onion and add the rest of the onion to the processor. Blend until smooth, adding 1 tablespoon of water, if needed, to thin out the mixture.

7. Season with salt (if using). Allow the salsa to cool completely in the refrigerator before serving.

APPENDIX

Paleo Snacks

It is often hardest to stick to a diet when hunger strikes. This appendix provides snack ideas to incorporate into the Paleo way of eating. Keep these snacks on hand, so when hunger strikes there is a healthy alternative within close reach. When consuming fruit, be sure to combine it with a little healthful fat or protein to prevent blood sugar levels from spiking.

- Endive spears or cucumber slices topped with 1 slice of cut-up smoked salmon
- Leftover chicken or other cooked meat, eaten plain or as a roll-up with Dijon mustard, avocado slices, and large lettuce leaves
- Handful of berries with 1 to 2 hard-boiled eggs
- 8 to 10 baby carrots or 1 small apple with 1 to 2 tablespoons unsalted nut butter
- 1 Nutty Fruit Bar (page 70)
- ¼ to ½ cup Chia Seed Pudding (page 138) with a sprinkling of berries and toasted unsalted nuts
- 1 fried or microwaved egg with 1 to 2 slices of tomato
- Bell pepper or jicama slices with quick guacamole: one-half avocado mashed with a squeeze of a lime wedge and minced jalapeño or serrano pepper
- Ants on a log: 5 celery sticks with 1 to 2 tablespoons unsalted almond butter, topped with goji berries or dried unsweetened cherries
- 1 to 2 pieces dried nitrate-free turkey or beef jerky
- Trail mix: 3 tablespoons dried unsweetened fruit with 3 tablespoons unsalted cashews, almonds, or other nuts
- 15 whole almonds with 1 to 2 hard-boiled eggs
- 1 egg and a handful of spinach stirred into 1 cup Chicken Broth (page 158)
- 3 or 4 pitted dates, each stuffed with 1 almond
- 1 to 2 Almond Butter Bites (page 143)

- Easy tuna salad: 3 ounces tuna packed in water, drained and mixed with ½ tablespoon Dijon mustard, 1 teaspoon oil, and juice of one-half lemon served with cucumber slices
- One-half chicken sausage link with ½ cup sliced, cooked sweet potato tossed in ½ tablespoon coconut oil
- 1 small apple with 1 to 2 tablespoons almond butter

Resources

Barclay, Alan W., Peter Petocz, Joanna McMillan-Price, Victoria M. Flood, Tania Prvan, Paul Mitchell, and Jennie C. Brand-Miller. "Glycemic Index, Glycemic Load and Chronic Disease Risk—A Meta-Analysis of Observational Studies." *American Journal of Clinical Nutrition* 87 (2008): 627–37. http://ajcn.nutrition.org/content/87/3/627.full.pdf.

Booth, Frank W., Manu V. Chakravarthy, and Espen E. Spangenburg. "Exercise and Gene Expression: Physiological Regulation of the Human Genome Through Physical Activity." *Journal of Physiology* 543 (June 2002): 399–411. doi:10.1113/jphysiol.2002.019265.

Cordain, Loren. "Published Research About the Paleo Diet." The Paleo Diet. Accessed January 8, 2014. http://thepaleodiet.com/published-research-about-the-paleo-diet/.

Cordain, Loren. *The Paleo Answer: 7 Days to Lose Weight, Feel Great, Stay Young.* New York: Houghton Mifflin Harcourt, 2012.

Cordain, Loren. *The Paleo Diet: Lose Weight and Get Healthy by Eating the Foods You Were Designed to Eat.* Rev. ed. New York: Houghton Mifflin Harcourt, 2013.

Cordain, Loren. "The Protein Debate: Dr. Loren Cordain and T. Colin Campbell." Catalyst Athletics. March 19, 2008. http://www.catalystathletics.com/articles/article.php?articleID=50.

Cordain, L., R. W. Gotshall, S. B. Eaton, and S. B. Eaton III. "Physical Activity, Energy Expenditure and Fitness: An Evolutionary Perspective." *International Journal of Sports Medicine* 19, no. 5 (July 1998): 328–35. http://thepaleodiet.com/wp-content/uploads/2012/04/Int-J-Sport-Article.pdf.

Lindeberg, S., T. Jönsson, Y. Granfeldt, E. Borgstrand, J. Soffman, K. Sjöström, and B. Ahrén. "A Palaeolithic Diet Improves Glucose Tolerance More Than a Mediterranean-Like Diet in Individuals with Ischaemic Heart Disease." *Diabetologia* 50, no. 9 (September 2007): 1795–1807. http://link.springer.com/article/10.1007%2Fs00125-007-0716-y.

Miller, Janette Brand, Neil Mann, and Loren Cordain. *Paleolithic Nutrition: What Did Our Ancestors Eat?* The Paleo Diet. Accessed January 8, 2014. http://thepaleodiet.com/wp-content/uploads/2012/04/chapter-3-Brand-Miller.pdf.

Wolf, Robb. *The Paleo Solution: The Original Human Diet*. Las Vegas: Victory Belt Publishing, 2010.